Dr. Dvir Levin | THE RIGHT TO CHOOSE

THE RIGHT TO CHOOSE

Self-published - Dr. Dvir Levin
Content editing, language editing, proofreading, typesetting, and production: Dr. Dvir Levin

Printed edition | 2026
ISBN for the English edition: 978-965-93397-0-9

THE RIGHT TO CHOOSE

Who Really Decides About Our Bodies?

The Revolution That Changed Medicine and Human Rights

Dr. Dvir Levin

English Edition | 2026

Author's Note

This book seeks to connect history, law, and practical experience within the healthcare system. It invites discussion, criticism, and deeper inquiry: the testimony of a patient or staff member may reveal a gap that a legal rule does not capture, while systematic data may correct an impression formed from a single case. The purpose of the book is not to set patients against healthcare professionals, but to propose a language that protects both - and the shared space in which care takes place.

Contents

Contents - continued

Foreword

This book addresses a question that appears simple only at first glance: when did the patient cease to be a person dependent on the healer's benevolence and professional skill and become a holder of rights vis-à-vis the physician, the institution, and the state? The answer is not found in a single date. It unfolds across ancient oaths, religious traditions, the rise of the hospital, the Nuremberg trials, the development of informed consent, rights movements, welfare states, and national legislation. At every stage, not only the language changed, but also the question of who is entitled to decide what is in the best interests of the person who is ill.

The title The Right to Choose emphasizes the transition from a patient who is the object of decisions to a person with a voice and a right to choose. Yet benevolence and rights are not enemies. Benevolence is the willingness to see the person beyond the minimum that is legally required, to remain at the bedside, to explain again, and to show humanity when curative treatment is no longer available. Benevolence alone, however, depends on the character of the person who holds power. A right seeks to guarantee a floor that is not reserved only for those who inspire sympathy, know someone in the system, or are able to fight for themselves. Conversely, a right without benevolence can become a form, a signature, and a cold transfer of information. Good medicine needs both languages.

The book places Israel at its center but does not stop there. The Patient's Rights Law, 5756-1996, was an important legal and conceptual achievement. It entrenched proper medical care, non-discrimination, informed consent, confidentiality, medical records, and the right to information. Yet the law was born within a public system that sometimes struggles to provide time, a bed, an appointment, or privacy. This gap does not prove that the law failed; it proves that law requires infrastructure. Rights are realized not only in the courtroom, but also in the corridor, the emergency department, the appointment line, and the transition from hospital to community care.

One of the book's sensitive themes is violence against healthcare staff. Public discussion sometimes raises the claim that patient empowerment and the language of 'I am entitled to this' weakened the physician's status and contributed to violence. The claim deserves examination, but it should not become a conclusion before alternative explanations are considered: workload, waiting, uncertainty, inequality, commercialization, misinformation, and a broader crisis of trust in authority. The book will show that changing expectations can be acknowledged without attributing to the law a causal relationship that has not been demonstrated, and that protecting staff does not require retreating from patients' rights.

The book is written for a broad audience: physicians and nurses, healthcare managers, legal professionals, students, policymakers, patients, and readers interested in the relationship among medicine, society, and human rights. It is not a legal guide for an individual case and does not replace professional advice. Its purpose is to offer a historical, legal, and comparative journey, identify tensions, and propose a model of rights with mutual responsibility. Each chapter moves among idea, institution, and case, because in healthcare a principle has little meaning if it does not reach the person at the moment it is needed.

Introduction: From Professional Duty to Human Right

The Central Question and the Guiding Argument

This book examines how patients' rights developed worldwide and in Israel, and especially how they should be assessed after evolving from moral principles into legal and institutional frameworks. Its central argument is that discussion of rights cannot stop at asking whether a particular rule exists in law; it must also examine who bears responsibility for implementing it, what resources are available, how a decision is explained, and how a failure can be corrected in time. Against this background, the book explores the tensions between autonomy and professional judgment, equality and allocation, and patient protection and staff safety, without assuming in advance that one value necessarily cancels out another.

The book distinguishes among three concepts. The first is medical ethics: the duties and values that guide professionals. The second is patients' rights: claims held by a person within the therapeutic encounter, such as information, consent, privacy, and dignity. The third is the right to health: the social obligation of the state to promote access, quality, and equality. The three concepts overlap but are not identical. A system may sustain devoted ethical practice without legal enforcement, protect consent within a system that is inaccessible, or entrench health in a constitution without guaranteeing privacy in the treatment room.

A further distinction is required between the existence of a right and the ability to exercise it. A legal document defines an expectation, but actual behavior is shaped by incentives, workload, hierarchy, organizational culture, and a person's ability to seek help. The proper measure, therefore, is not only the wording of the law, but the proportion of people who can understand their rights and use them without paying an unreasonable price. Strong rights are not the enemy of an efficient system; they require the system to explain its limits, measure its performance, and correct itself.

Method of Inquiry and Comparative Framework

The book is based on the collection, reading, and comparison of historical, legal, and institutional sources. It combines foundational documents, legislation and case law, policy reviews, and descriptions of healthcare systems. The sources include the Hippocratic Oath and the medical tradition of Maimonides; the Nuremberg Code, the Declaration of Helsinki, and the Belmont Report; instruments of the United Nations and the World Health Organization; Israeli laws and judicial decisions; and official documents concerning the countries discussed. Bioethical and sociological literature is used to interpret the gap between written rules and actual behavior.

For legal claims, priority is given to statutory texts, judicial decisions, and official documents; for descriptions of systems and policy, priority is given to publications of governments, international organizations, and public research bodies; and scholarly literature is used for framing, interpretation, and comparison. Where a secondary source summarizes law or policy, it is read alongside the primary source whenever that source is accessible. References are selected as anchor sources rather than as an exhaustive list, with emphasis on implementation mechanisms and on the gap between a formal rule and its practical use.

Countries are compared along analytical dimensions rather than ranked. The analysis considers the source of the right, organization of financing, access to services, rights within the clinical encounter, complaint mechanisms, and the relationship between patients and staff. This method avoids the simplistic conclusion that a country with a broad constitutional provision necessarily offers better protection than one relying on statutory arrangements. It also makes it possible to identify institutional substitutes: a right may be enforced through a court, a regulator, an ombudsman, public insurance, or a combination of these mechanisms.

The method of inquiry seeks to avoid two opposite errors: inferring causation from striking cases alone, and erasing human experience merely because it does not appear in a database. The argument therefore relies on triangulation among historical and legal documents, professional literature, policy data, and institutional description. The comparison does not rank countries; it asks which mechanisms turn a written right into a practical capability.

Limits of the Discussion

The book does not claim to present a new empirical database or a complete mapping of incidents of violence and complaints. Data in different countries are collected under different definitions and methods, and the volume of reporting is affected by awareness and reporting practices. Claims about trends and causation are therefore framed cautiously. Likewise, the terms 'the West,' 'Asia,' and 'Africa' conceal enormous diversity; the countries selected are comparative cases and do not represent entire continents.

Another limitation concerns the nature of the sources. Law and policy change, and the discussion should not be read as though institutional arrangements were frozen in time. Where a historical source is disputed, such as the attribution of certain texts to Maimonides, the discussion addresses the tradition and its influence rather than asserting a definitive philological conclusion.

These limits require a distinction between normative claims about what ought to be and evidence about what actually occurs. A full assessment of the implementation of rights and violence within the healthcare system would require uniform quantitative data, interviews, complaint analysis, and observation of work processes. This book offers an interpretive and comparative framework for critically reading the existing material.

Structure of the Book

Part One presents the global roots: ancient ethics, Nuremberg and Helsinki, and the autonomy revolution. Part Two turns to Israel - from institutional medicine, through social and constitutional catalysts, to an analysis of the Patient's Rights Law. Part Three examines the post-law reality: resources, quality, access, violence, and the claim of a boomerang effect. Part Four compares Israel with Brazil and Bolivia; the United States and Canada; China, Japan, Thailand, and Malaysia; Nigeria and South Africa; and the United Kingdom and Germany. The final part offers a synthesis and proposed reforms.

The historical sequence makes it possible to see that patients' rights were not imposed on medicine from outside, but developed in response to recurring problems across different periods: dependence on expert knowledge, use of the person as a means, concealment of information, discrimination, and scarcity. Each stage added a layer of protection while also exposing new limits of law and professional practice. The book therefore does not present a sharp transition from paternalism to autonomy, but an ongoing process of limiting power, expanding voice, and building mechanisms of correction.

The comparison among countries complements the historical perspective. It shows that no institutional model is perfect and that the same right may be realized through legislation, public insurance, a regulator, an ombudsman, or a combination of mechanisms. The central question is not which country formulated the most impressive declaration, but which combinations of financing, professional practice, participation, and enforcement allow a vulnerable person to receive fair care while also giving staff the conditions to work safely and responsibly. The book may be read from beginning to end, but each part is also designed to stand on its own: as historical background, an Israeli analysis, an international comparison, or a tool for professional and managerial thinking.

Part One: The Historical Roots of Medical Ethics and Patients' Rights Worldwide

Part One seeks to show that patients' rights did not appear at a single moment and were not born solely from modern legislation. They grew out of a long encounter among traditions of professional benevolence, moral duties, scientific authority, historical trauma, and new conceptions of human dignity. The central distinction is between ethics, which defines what a physician ought to do, and rights-based discourse, which gives the patient an institutional and legal claim against the physician, the hospital, and the state.

Chapter One: From Antiquity to the Early Modern Period - Oath, Benevolence, and Paternalism

Opening Dilemma

A patient is hospitalized in an internal-medicine ward after a difficult night. In the morning, a senior physician enters with two residents and a group of students. The physician says, "We will examine you together," and begins presenting the case. The patient hesitates, pulls the blanket closer, and avoids eye contact, but does not say no. Formally, no objection has been voiced; humanly, several signs suggest that the consent is not freely given. One short and direct question - Are you comfortable with the students remaining, and is it clear that your care will not be affected if you prefer otherwise? - changes the balance of power. If the examination is intimate, it is appropriate to limit attendance in advance rather than placing on the patient the burden of asking a group that has already entered to leave.

Before the patient was a bearer of rights, the patient was the object of a duty. Ancient medical ethics placed important limits on the healer's power, but its center of gravity lay in the character and obligations of the professional rather than in the patient's independent rights.

1. Ancient Medicine Between the Sacred, Craft, and Knowledge

In ancient societies, there was no sharp separation among medicine, religion, philosophy, and social order. The healer was seen as someone mediating among the body, fate, and the community, and therefore possessed authority far broader than that of a modern professional service provider. Historically, in

Mesopotamia and Egypt, therapeutic instructions appeared alongside incantations, rituals, and rules of responsibility. In classical Greece, a tradition developed that sought to explain illness through observation and natural causation, even though it did not completely abandon the world of the gods. The emergence of medical schools created an early professional identity and a demand for controlled transmission of knowledge.

At the organizational level, care took place in the home, in temples, on the battlefield, or at the bedside of a wealthy person. There was no public institution with a duty of equality, and no orderly system of licensing, appeal, or complaint. Personal dependence on the healer and on the family shaped power relations in which the patient possessed little information and few alternatives. The contrast, for example, between the Code of Hammurabi, which in some situations set compensation and punishment for healers, and the Hippocratic tradition illustrates two early forms of oversight: external accountability imposed by authority versus internal discipline within the profession.

At the same time, the very existence of rules was not equivalent to patients' rights. A rule could protect professional order, the reputation of a school, or the status of the head of the household without recognizing the sick person as an autonomous bearer of wishes and claims. This distinction later reappeared in Israeli history as well: for decades there were professional norms and a strong sense of medical mission, but no central instrument defining an independent patient right to information, confidentiality, consent, and dignity.

The first lesson is that professional morality is essential but insufficient. Modern protection also requires external mechanisms: legislation, documentation, review, access to information, and a practical route to redress when professional duties are not fulfilled.

2. The Hippocratic Oath: An Ethic of the Healer, Not a Charter of Rights

The Hippocratic Oath was revolutionary in establishing self-restraint, confidentiality, and a commitment to avoid harm, but it was written in the first person of the physician rather than in the language of the patient's rights. Historically, the Hippocratic text, associated with a tradition dating to the fifth and fourth centuries BCE, dealt with teacher-student relations, therapeutic boundaries, prohibitions, and conduct in the patient's home. Over the centuries it was translated, edited, and adapted to different cultures, and at times was attributed a uniformity that never existed in practice (Edelstein, 1943).

In practice, the oath strengthened the physician's identity as a member of a moral community. It built trust through an internal promise: not to exploit access to the body and the home, to keep secrets, and to act for the patient's benefit. Enforcement, however, depended mainly on conscience, reputation, and peers. Confidentiality is a good example of the complexity. It protects the patient, yet in the oath it appears as the physician's duty of silence. Only in a later legal world did confidentiality also become the patient's right to control information concerning them.

This approach, however, creates benevolent paternalism: the physician is expected to seek the patient's good, but is also the one who defines what that good is. When professional judgment conflicts with the patient's wishes, the text contains no systematic mechanism for preferring the person's choice. The language of oath and vocation remained influential in medical education in Israel as well. The Patient's Rights Law did not abolish that tradition; it added another layer - professional duties that can be translated into rights, procedures, and legal review.

A contemporary system need not choose between oath and law. Organizational culture needs internal ethics so that law does not become an empty form, while law is needed so that ethics does not remain dependent solely on whether a particularly good person happens to be in the room.

3. Maimonides: Medicine, Humility, and Human Dignity

The medical writings of Maimonides present a rich model of the learned, cautious physician who is conscious of the limits of knowledge. In this sense, the tradition approaches modern ideas of dignity, even though it does not formulate autonomy in the liberal sense. Maimonides worked in the twelfth century as a physician, jurist, and philosopher in a multicultural Jewish-Islamic world. His writings addressed nutrition, hygiene, prevention, physical and mental illness, and ways of life. He emphasized looking at the whole person rather than only at the diseased organ (Rosner, 1998).

Institutionally, the Maimonidean physician possesses broad knowledge but is not omnipotent. The physician must study, remain current, consider the circumstances of each individual, and avoid arrogance. This is especially important in a modern system in which technological expertise can create the illusion that a clinically possible decision is always the ethically correct one. The tradition associated with the "Physician's Prayer," even where the question of its precise authorship is debated, expresses an ideal of patience, love of humanity, and recognition that rich and poor deserve equal attention. That ideal approaches the principle of non-discrimination.

Compassion, however, is not the same as partnership. A physician may be humble and humane and still decide for the patient. The move from a moral relationship to autonomy requires recognition that even a decision the physician considers mistaken may be the legitimate decision of a competent person. In Israeli discourse, which combines Jewish tradition, liberal democracy, and social solidarity, Maimonides can serve as a bridge. He makes it possible to discuss human dignity not merely as a Western legal import but also as part of a local tradition of responsibility and humility.

The contemporary application is medical education that combines communication skills, awareness of limitations, listening, and social responsibility. Rights are not realized when a patient receives a form; they are realized when the team is genuinely prepared to hear the patient's story and, when appropriate, revise its decision.

4. The Hospital and the Birth of Clinical Authority

The rise of the modern hospital and clinical science greatly expanded medicine's ability to save lives, but it also widened the gap between those who know, document, and decide and the person whose body becomes the object of examination. Historically, from the early modern period through the nineteenth century, hospitals evolved from charitable institutions and shelters for the poor into centers of teaching, research, and treatment. Pathology, anatomy, the laboratory, and statistics transformed the patient's bedside into a site for the production of knowledge.

At the institutional level, the new structure required discipline: visiting hours, hierarchy, documentation, division into departments, and uniform rules. The patient gained access to specialists and technology but lost some control over environment, time, and information. Medical language became more precise and also less accessible. The clinical examination in which a group of students gathers around a bed illustrates this duality. It allows the training of generations of physicians, but without consent, privacy, and explanation it can turn a person into a sign, a finding, or an "interesting case."

The reality is even more complex: an institution is not merely a collection of professionals. Even an empathetic physician works within a system of queues, pressure, shortages, and performance indicators. Patients' rights must therefore apply to the organization itself - not only to the caregiver's intentions, but also to the design of the physical space and the care process. Hospitals in Israel inherited European traditions, charitable institutions, military medicine, and a public health-fund model. The organizational culture that grew within them gave substantial weight to expertise and the national mission and, at times, less weight to the voice of the individual.

Recognition of institutional rights requires physical privacy, linguistic accessibility, an explanation of bedside teaching, the ability to refuse the presence of trainees, and complaint systems that do not depend on the very person the patient fears.

5. The Paternalistic Model: Advantages, Risks, and Survivals

Medical paternalism is not simply a dark relic. It arose from genuine dependence on knowledge and rescue. The problem begins when professional dependence is presented as justification for denying voice, information, and choice. Historically, for centuries the information gap between physician and patient was almost absolute. In situations of pain, anxiety, and danger to life, the assumption that the physician would decide could seem natural and even humane. Families sometimes asked that serious diagnoses be concealed, and physicians feared that information would harm the patient or destroy hope.

In practice, paternalism can be soft, when the team guides choice while leaving room for decision, or hard, when treatment is imposed or information withheld. It can be temporary, in an emergency or during incapacity, or routine, as part of a culture in which questions are treated as an interruption. A decision not to tell a patient about a malignancy in order to "preserve hope," for example, illustrates both the intention to benefit and the cost. Without information, a person cannot arrange personal affairs, choose treatment, seek a second opinion, or decide how to live the time that remains.

At the other extreme, complete autonomy is also a fiction. Patients depend on explanation, recommendation, family, and resources. The alternative to paternalism is therefore not abandonment of the patient in front of a menu of options, but shared decision-making that acknowledges inequality of knowledge and power and seeks to reduce it. In Israel, remnants of paternalism remain visible in phrases such as "You don't need to know" or "Sign here." Conversely, fear of litigation can produce a technical and overwhelming discharge of information. Both situations miss the purpose of the law: genuine understanding and meaningful choice (O'Neill, 2002; Mol, 2008).

The challenge is justified and narrowly tailored paternalism: intervention only where there is a clear clinical and legal basis, for the shortest possible period, with documentation, consultation, reconsideration, and respect for the person's prior wishes insofar as they can be known.

Clinical Application: Bedside Teaching as a Test of Legitimate Authority

The entry of trainees into the room of a hospitalized person concentrates, in a single moment, the tension among professional education, hierarchy, privacy, and consent. Clear working rules are required before entry, during the examination, and after any change in the scope of permission.

Consent That Is Never Spoken Aloud

A patient may remain silent because they agree, but also because they are tired, embarrassed, or afraid that refusal will affect their care. The absence of objection is therefore not enough. Permission should be requested before the group enters, in direct language, together with a clear statement that choosing otherwise will not change the professional care provided.

The team needs a graduated model of authorization: observation only, conversation, limited examination, performance of a procedure, or photography for teaching purposes. Each move to a higher level requires appropriate consent. This graduated model allows the patient to choose without being forced into a binary yes-or-no answer, and teaches the trainee that access to another person's body does not automatically accompany professional status.

What to Measure and How to Correct

An institution that wishes to evaluate itself should not merely count consent forms. A short periodic sample can examine whether the purpose of the trainees' presence was explained, whether the patient knew that refusal was possible, whether privacy was preserved, and whether a complaint received a timely response. This can be combined with brief patient interviews, observation of staff, and review of situations in which discomfort arose.

A record showing one hundred percent signed consent forms may conceal a routine in which no one feels free to say no. By contrast, a certain rate of refusals is not necessarily failure; it may indicate that the option was presented credibly. The review should also include staff. Do trainees know how to ask permission? Is a nurse allowed to raise a concern without being treated as obstructing teaching? Does the physician have enough time to explain?

If policy places the entire burden on one individual during periods of heavy workload, it will quickly erode. One possible solution is a short and consistent ritual at the beginning of the examination: introduce those present, distinguish treatment from teaching, and ask explicitly for permission. Sensitive examinations require a private conversation. The simpler and clearer the process, the more likely it is to be maintained even on a busy ward.

In Israel, a uniform national principle is appropriate, but not a single formula for every situation. Guidance should make clear that refusal of a presence not necessary for treatment does not affect entitlement to care; that consent can be changed; and that intimate examinations require heightened caution. Hospitals can adapt the explanation to the population, language, and type of department. Oversight should focus on the result - understanding, privacy, and the ability to refuse - and not merely on the existence of a written procedure. In this way, a common minimum standard can be preserved without turning the clinical encounter into a lengthy legal ceremony.

Capacity, Support, and Real-Time Decision-Making

An emergency sharpens the tension between the need to act and the duty to respect choice. When a person is unconscious, the team may provide life-saving treatment in accordance with law and clinical necessity. Once the condition stabilizes, however, the exception narrows. The team must return to the person, explain what was done, and seek consent for continued treatment. The emergency exception is not a general authorization for everything that is convenient to perform during hospitalization. Documentation of urgency, alternatives, and the point at which the conversation was renewed helps distinguish necessity from habit. The important institutional principle is that an exception born of urgency must be time-limited and must end when the conditions that justified it disappear.

After stabilization, responsibility shifts from deciding in the person's place to restoring the person to the conversation and to shared decision-making. The systematic discussion of capacity - how understanding is assessed, how decision-making is supported, and what weight should be given to family - appears in Chapter Three.

Benevolence, Apology, and Repair

When a boundary has been crossed, the institution's response determines whether the harm deepens. An apology does not replace an inquiry, but it recognizes the person's experience and reduces the need to prove that they were harmed. The institution should explain what is known, what will be examined, and when an answer will be provided. If the procedure itself was unclear, the correction should be systemic and not limited to a conversation with the employee. In appropriate cases, the patient can be invited to contribute to designing the change without making the patient responsible for repairing the system.

The connection between benevolence and rights becomes especially visible here. Benevolence is the willingness to listen beyond the minimum; a right is the guarantee that listening does not depend on the character of the individual caregiver. A good system embeds humane conduct in a flexible procedure: time for explanation, the option to refuse, a clear address for complaints, and a respectful response. It does not seek to turn every encounter into a lawsuit; it seeks to create conditions in which expertise can operate without silencing the person. This is the transition from the good healer to the worthy institution.

Teaching the Trainee to Ask Permission

Asking permission is a clinical skill that can be taught and assessed. The trainee should introduce themselves, explain what they are asking to do, recognize signs of discomfort, and withdraw respectfully. Assessment can include not only accuracy of the examination, but also the quality of the explanation and the trainee's response to refusal.

A responsible teaching institution should create alternatives: simulation, standardized patients, volunteer pools, and rotation planning that does not depend on one particular patient. When alternatives exist, a patient's refusal becomes a real choice rather than a threat to the training of the next generation.

Exceeding the Scope of Permission: Stop, Clarify, Repair

A patient agrees to the presence of one student during a routine examination. During the encounter, two additional trainees join, and the physician decides to extend the examination to a more intimate area. This is not a technical detail: it changes both the number of people present and the nature of the contact. The examination must therefore stop and renewed permission must be requested. The original consent cannot be assumed to cover every possible development.

An appropriate response begins with immediate recognition of the change: introduce those present, briefly explain the need, and offer a choice among proceeding, limiting, or postponing the examination. If the patient hesitates, the default should be to limit the encounter. Afterward, the departure from the original permission and the corrective action should be documented, not in order to assign automatic blame to the trainee, but to identify whether a crowded teaching schedule, lack of briefing, or a departmental norm produced a quiet expansion of permission.

Systemic correction may include clearly marking the scope of consent, a short briefing before teaching rounds, and enabling every staff member to stop the encounter without fear of hierarchy. Consent then becomes not a one-time gesture but a working rule responsive to changing circumstances.

The Profession Organizes: Licensing, Guilds, and the Boundaries of Competence

Between the ancient healer and the modern physician lies a long process of professional organization. Cities, universities, and rulers began to define who was permitted to practice medicine, how training would be assessed, and what counted as conduct outside the boundaries of the profession. Early licensing was not primarily designed to protect patient autonomy; it sought to maintain order, distinguish knowledgeable practitioners from impostors, and protect the status of professional groups. Nevertheless, the very possibility of withdrawing permission to practice created a form of public accountability that did not depend solely on the healer's personal reputation.

Guilds and universities also had an exclusionary side. They determined who could study, which traditions counted as legitimate knowledge, and which folk healers were pushed to the margins. Women, midwives, and minority groups continued to care for people in the community, sometimes without institutional recognition. This history shows that professional standards can improve safety while also narrowing diversity and local knowledge. The modern licensing question is therefore not merely whether the professional passed an examination, but how the system assesses continuing competence, handles complaints, and enables correction before further harm occurs.

As hospitals expanded, licensing became multilayered: the state grants a basic license, the organization defines clinical privileges, and the department supervises actual practice. This mechanism matters to patients' rights because it connects general qualification with a specific act. A licensed physician is not automatically authorized to perform every procedure, and a trainee does not act without supervision. Patients' rights therefore depend not only on the character of the clinician but also on the quality of the system that defines boundaries, documents deviations, and updates privileges.

The modern idea of professional competence also adds a duty to learn. Medical knowledge changes, and a treatment once accepted may later prove ineffective or harmful. An organization that relies only on a historical certificate is not fulfilling its duty. Periodic assessment, simulation, peer feedback, and learning from adverse events transform licensing from a one-time document into a living protection mechanism.

The Emergence of Nursing and the Continuous Voice at the Bedside

The history of patients' rights is not only the history of physicians and law. The development of professional nursing created a role that remains beside the patient over time, notices small changes, and knows the gap between a medical order and the practical ability to carry it out. A nurse is not merely the executor of a decision; the nurse mediates information, identifies pain, hears reservations, and can raise an alarm when a formal process does not reflect genuine understanding.

This role developed gradually and often within a rigid hierarchy. Nursing traditions emphasized discipline, cleanliness, and order, but also observation, presence, and protection of the vulnerable. When the nurse was completely subordinate to the physician, the ability to stop an action or raise doubt was limited. The professionalization of nursing, independent training, and ethical codes expanded the possibility of treating safety and dignity as shared team responsibilities.

In bedside teaching, nursing has a particularly important role. A nurse may recognize that a patient agreed politely while tensing the body or avoiding eye contact. A sound organizational culture gives the nurse permission to ask again, to request that the number of people present be reduced, and to explain to trainees that consent can change during the encounter. This creates an internal balancing mechanism that does not depend on a later complaint.

The broader lesson is that rights are not protected by a single office-holder. They depend on a network of eyes, voices, and authorities. When every team member understands their responsibility and is able to speak even in the presence of a senior professional, clinical authority becomes safer, not weaker.

The Clinical Record and Turning the Person into a "Case"

The expansion of medical documentation made continuity, comparison, and research possible, but it also changed how the system sees the person. The record classifies signs, illnesses, and decisions, and at times pushes aside the story that does not fit a structured field. A patient may come to be seen through a previous diagnosis, a documented behavior, or a sentence written in a context that no longer exists.

In the nineteenth century, documentation primarily served the physician and the hospital. In a rights-based world, it also became a source of information for the patient and a tool of review. This change requires distinguishing factual description from interpretation, identifying the source of information, and correcting an error without erasing history. It also demands caution in the use of words that may follow a person for years and alter the attitude of staff who have never met that person.

In a teaching institution, the record can turn a case into educational material detached from the person. Case presentation should minimize unnecessary details, protect identity, and remind trainees that every data point belongs to the life of a person who holds rights. Good documentation is not only accurate; it is proportionate, respectful, and capable of being explained.

From the Poor Patient to the User of a Public Service

Early hospitals relied heavily on charity, religion, and philanthropy. The recipient was sometimes seen as owing gratitude and therefore not entitled to demand much. The transition to a public system changed the relationship: the service is funded by public resources, and the individual is not a guest dependent on the institution's goodwill. Every person is entitled to a minimum standard of care, information, and dignity even when they do not evoke sympathy and cannot give anything in return.

The change does not abolish solidarity or benevolence. It transfers them from personal generosity to shared responsibility. Precisely because the system is public, it must explain its constraints and allocate resources in a manner that can be justified to everyone who depends on it.

Pharmacy and the Separation of Prescribing from Dispensing

The development of pharmacy as a distinct profession altered the distribution of power in medicine. When the same person diagnosed, prescribed, prepared, and sold a medicine, there was almost no external mechanism to check dosage, suitability, or financial incentive. Separating these functions created another point of control: the prescription became a document that could be read, questioned, and cross-checked against another body of professional knowledge.

The pharmacist occupies a unique position because the encounter occurs after the medical decision has already been made but before treatment actually begins. The pharmacist can identify duplication, an interaction, a financial difficulty, or a gap between the instruction and the patient's ability to use the treatment at home. This role is not competition with the physician; it is protection against errors that can arise in the transition from diagnosis to prescription, dispensing, and adherence.

Professional separation alone is not enough. If the pharmacist lacks access to relevant information, time for conversation, or a rapid way to contact the clinic, the checkpoint becomes merely technical. A modern system should define what information is required, how an intervention is documented, and what happens when disagreement arises. The history of the professions thus shows that the relative independence of different professionals can strengthen shared responsibility and give the patient more than one address for a question.

Anatomy, Body Donation, and Consent After Death

The study of anatomy has historically illustrated a different kind of gap between the needs of professional training and the status of the person. A deceased body is not a patient who can refuse in real time, but neither is it material without identity. The ways in which bodies were obtained for study - at times from prisoners, poor people, or individuals who had not consented - show how scientific benefit can conceal an unequal social distribution of burdens. Medical education requires access to the human body, but that need alone does not create an institutional right to use it.

Informed body donation changes the basis of legitimacy. During life, a person chooses whether to donate and receives information about the purposes of use, the duration of retention, possible research, commemoration, and final disposition. Consent that is too general may blur important distinctions among basic teaching, photography, technology development, and sharing with another institution. It is therefore preferable to offer graduated choices and document limitations set by the donor rather than assume that one donation authorizes every future use.

The family also has a legitimate human interest, but it should not be turned into the owner of a clearly expressed wish. When the donor's decision conflicts with the family's preference, a process is needed that respects the commitment made to the donor while explaining to the family what will be done. Early transparency reduces disputes: who will make contact after death, whether there will be a memorial ceremony, when remains will be returned, and whether consent may be withdrawn before death.

A teaching institution should teach respectful conduct even when no living patient is in the room. Anonymous presentation, restrictions on photography, information security, and non-degrading language are part of professional practice. A memorial ceremony is not a substitute for procedure, but it reminds the trainee that knowledge was received from a person who placed trust in the institution. In this way, body donation becomes an intergenerational partnership rather than a hidden continuation of a tradition in which the vulnerable supplied the material for learning.

Operational Map for Respectful Clinical Teaching

Decision Point	Preferred Arrangement	Responsible Party	Control Indicator
Before entry	Request permission in private and clarify that refusal will not affect care	Responsible physician	The patient knows who is entering and why
Scope of presence	Choice among observation, limited examination, or non-participation	Clinical instructor	The number of people present matches the patient's choice
Sensitive examination	Explicit consent, option of a support person, and necessary limitation	Person performing the examination	The procedure is not expanded without renewed permission
Recognizing discomfort	Stop and ask again even without an explicit "no"	Every staff member in the room	Hesitation leads to clarification, not pressure
After a boundary is exceeded	Explanation, apology, documentation, and procedural correction	Department head	A timely response and a change that can be audited

Respectful clinical teaching does not rest on the assumption that hospitalization includes surrender of control over the body. It is designed so that the patient can determine the extent of participation, and the trainee learns that asking permission is a professional skill. In such a structure, refusal is not a disruption of the teaching program but a fact that the institution must be able to accommodate.

Chapter Two: The Twentieth-Century Breaking Point - Experimentation, Law, and Informed Consent

Opening Dilemma

A patient with a rare disease comes to a physician she has known for years. He offers her participation in a study in which he is the principal investigator and says that the new treatment 'may be the best hope available.' The patient does not ask about alternatives because she is afraid of disappointing him. Formally, she can be given a detailed form; ethically, an additional separation is required. A person who is not part of the research team can explain the options, allow time for consultation, and make sure that the patient knows the therapeutic relationship will continue even if she refuses. The greater the dependence on the physician, the stronger the need for a consent pathway that does not rely on that physician alone. Financial incentives also require careful distinction.

Science lost its presumption of moral innocence.

The atrocities of human experimentation and the trials that followed the Second World War transformed consent from a secondary moral idea into an explicit principle limiting scientific and state power.

1. When Medicine Served the State Against the Individual

The twentieth century demonstrated that medical education, advanced research, and the language of public health do not guarantee morality; they can become mechanisms of coercion, selection, and destruction. Eugenic doctrines, scientific racism, and bureaucratic authority preceded Nazism and existed in various countries. The Nazi regime carried them to the extreme in forced sterilization, killing, and brutal experiments on prisoners and groups designated as unworthy.

Within the system, evil did not arise only from sadistic individuals. It rested on forms, committees, funding, hierarchy, and professional language that removed the victim from view. When an institution defines a person as research material or a biological burden, private conscience struggles to stop the machinery. Experiments involving cold, pressure, infections, and drugs in the camps illustrated a complete violation of consent and the prohibition on causing harm. The mere use of the word 'experiment' does not confer scientific or moral legitimacy on an act.

The lesson, however, is not that every modern study can be compared with those atrocities, but that protective duties must be built in from the outset. Reliance on investigators' intentions and future benefit is insufficient when participants are dependent, coerced, or vulnerable. In Israel, this lesson carries particular historical weight. Memory of the Holocaust contributed to sensitivity to human dignity, but also to strengthening state and medical institutions that were perceived as protectors of life. The tension between these two movements accompanies local rights discourse.

Modern safeguards must include an independent ethics committee, risk-benefit assessment, fair participant selection, revocable consent, transparency, and documentation. Scientific approval alone is not enough for research that fails to respect the person.

2. The Doctors' Trial and the Nuremberg Code

The Nuremberg Code stated clearly that voluntary consent is an essential condition of research involving human beings and shifted the source of legitimacy from the scientist to the participating individual. Historically, in 1947, as part of the judgment in the Doctors' Trial, ten principles for permissible research were formulated. The first held that the voluntary consent of the human subject is absolutely essential; the remaining principles addressed social value, scientific foundation, avoidance of suffering, proportionality of risk, investigator competence, and the right to terminate participation (United States v. Brandt, 1947).

Institutionally, the Code was not a binding international treaty in the ordinary sense, but it became a cornerstone. Its importance lay in its clarity: free will cannot be replaced by a claim that research benefits humanity or that the investigator knows better. For example, the requirement of legal capacity and understanding of participation reveals a problem that remains with us today: how can children, people with cognitive impairments, or patients in emergencies be included without exploiting them, while also not excluding them entirely from the possible benefits of research?

Nevertheless, the Nuremberg Code was sometimes regarded as too absolute for clinical research because medicine also involves people who are unable to consent. The later response was not abandonment of the principle but the construction of alternative safeguards, legal representatives, and risk minimization. In Israel, Israeli law distinguishes between treatment and research and uses Helsinki committees. Yet the same question stands in both fields: is consent a formal event of signing, or a communicative process in which a genuine opportunity to ask questions and refuse is provided?

The Code should be read not only as a historical document but also as a warning against expanding exceptions. Emergencies, economic dependence, and therapeutic hope require heightened caution because they can turn an apparent choice into consent that is not truly free.

3. From Consent to Research to Consent to Treatment

The concept of 'informed consent' developed gradually in clinical law: from a prohibition on touching a person without permission to a duty to provide information relevant to choice. Historically, early American decisions, including Schloendorff in 1914, emphasized a person's right to determine what shall be done with their body. In 1957, the term informed consent appeared in Salgo, and later Canterbury v. Spence strengthened a standard centered on information that a reasonable patient would regard as material (Faden & Beauchamp, 1986).

In clinical reality, this represented a profound change in the law of negligence and battery. Treatment without any consent may amount to bodily interference, while treatment provided after partial consent but without adequate disclosure is examined as a failure of information and of the decision-making process. Suppose a procedure was performed skillfully and succeeded, but a material risk was not explained. The older tradition tended to say there was no medical harm and therefore no wrong. The autonomy approach argues that the person was denied the opportunity to choose, and that this too constitutes an injury.

When the principle is translated into practice, how much information is enough? Listing every remote risk can overwhelm the patient, while excessive filtering returns power to the physician. The answer is material information adapted to the individual, including alternatives, chances of success, risks of non-treatment, and room for personal preferences. In Israel, Israeli case law preceding the statute, and later section 13 of the Patient's Rights Law, adopted the duty of informed consent. The Daaka decision also recognized, in appropriate cases, infringement of autonomy as an independent head of damage (CA 2781/93 Daaka v. Carmel Hospital, 1999).

High-quality consent requires time, understandable language, cultural adaptation, the possibility of a second opinion, and documentation of the conversation rather than only the signature. A form may be evidence, but it is not a substitute for the process.

4. The Declaration of Helsinki and the Medical Profession as Gatekeeper

The Declaration of Helsinki sought to translate the lessons of Nuremberg into the continuing world of medical research and to impose on physicians a responsibility that does not disappear even where local law is more permissive. The World Medical Association adopted the Declaration in 1964 and has revised it many times, most recently in 2024. The changes reflect developments in multicenter research, placebo use, trial registration, publication of results, databases, vulnerability, and global fairness (World Medical Association, 2024).

In the clinical-research arena, the Declaration requires a protocol, independent ethics review, risk assessment, protection of vulnerable groups, and consent. It also recognizes that a physician-investigator may face a conflict between the patient's welfare and the goal of producing knowledge. For example, in a study offered to a poor population in a low-resource country, a signature is not enough. One must ask whether the community bears the risks but will benefit from the results, whether alternative treatment is accessible, and whether participation results from a lack of real medical alternatives.

Still, a professional declaration is not global law, and its various versions have generated controversy. Yet its flexibility is also an advantage: it allows the medical community to set an ethical threshold above the local minimum and to update that threshold in response to new technologies. In Israel, the term "Helsinki Committee" became part of the institutional language of research. The challenge is to prevent the committee from becoming a bureaucratic stamp and to preserve its role as an independent reviewer of science, fairness, and consent.

The 2024 revision strengthens the need for transparency, fair inclusion, and protection of vulnerable participants. Institutions should publish results, including negative results, manage conflicts of interest, and formulate participant information in non-promotional language.

5. Persistent Failure: Tuskegee, Institutions, and Dependence

Post-war documents did not prevent further abuses. The Tuskegee case and other studies showed that racism, institutional secrecy, and social dependence can bypass well-known ethical codes. Historically, the Tuskegee syphilis study ran in the United States from 1932 to 1972, and even after penicillin became accepted treatment, participants did not receive adequate care. Exposure of the case contributed to the National Research Act and the Belmont Report.

At the institutional level, the Belmont Report articulated three principles: respect for persons, beneficence, and justice. The principle of justice expanded the discussion beyond consent: even a person who agrees may be exploited if their group is selected because of its vulnerability and does not share in the benefits of the research. The case illustrates that distrust among minority groups is not necessarily ignorance. At times it is the collective memory of institutions that promised care but used people as means (National Commission, 1979).

The issue is complex, however: an institutional response can become so burdensome that beneficial research is blocked. It is therefore necessary to distinguish bureaucracy from protection: every requirement should be connected to risk, vulnerability, and the participant's degree of control. In Israel too, some groups have experienced discriminatory treatment or coercive attempts by institutions. A sensitive consent process must acknowledge history and gaps in trust rather than interpreting every expression of suspicion as a patient's failure to understand.

Building trust requires public participation, community representation, information about results, a mechanism for compensation for harm, and access to care after the study. Trust is not something the public is asked to provide; it is the result of proper conduct over time.

Research Governance: Protection Throughout the Life Cycle of a Clinical Study

Protection of a research participant does not end with the signing of a form. It begins with selection of the research question and population, continues through recruitment, monitoring, and reporting of adverse events, and ends only after arrangements have been made for data use, care following harm, and access to the results.

Separating the Roles of Treatment and Research

When the treating physician is also the principal investigator, a medical recommendation and an invitation to research are heard in the same voice. The patient may understand the study to be the recommended treatment or may fear that refusal will damage the relationship. Effective protection is not a blanket ban on dual roles but a division of tasks: a staff member who is not dependent on recruitment explains the study, the alternatives, and the option to withdraw, while the treating physician clarifies what care will continue outside the protocol.

Information about a possible therapeutic benefit must also be separated from marketing language. Phrases such as "the best hope" require disclosure of uncertainty, of the purpose of the study, and of the possibility that the intervention will not help. Documentation of the conversation should reflect the questions asked and the alternatives discussed, not merely delivery of the form.

When a treating physician recruits for research, payment may compensate for time, travel, and inconvenience, but an especially high amount may transform a risk that a person would otherwise reject into an option they cannot economically afford to refuse. There is no single formula for every situation; the participant's circumstances, level of risk, and whether payment is presented as compensation or as a reward must be examined. The ethics committee should review recruitment materials and advertising language, not only the scientific protocol. Terms such as "breakthrough treatment" may mislead even if they are not narrowly false.

Oversight Throughout the Research Life Cycle

Initial approval is not enough. A study may change when adverse events emerge, new information is discovered, or withdrawal rates are higher than expected. Quality oversight examines protocol deviations, complaints, harms not reported on time, and the reasons people leave. A withdrawal rate is not necessarily a failure; sometimes it shows that participants understand their right to withdraw. The question is whether those who left received continuing care, whether pressure was applied, and whether the institution learned from the reasons they gave. Global research adds a question of justice. Before a study begins, it is necessary to ask whether the research question is relevant to the community's needs, what will remain after funding ends, and whether there will be access to the product if it proves beneficial. Otherwise, the institution extracts knowledge from vulnerability without strengthening those who bore the cost. Databases, genetics, and artificial intelligence challenge the model of consent as a one-time event.

A sample collected for one purpose may be used years later to answer a question that could not have been anticipated. Genetic risk can affect family members, and a data breach can harm an entire group. Continuous governance is therefore required: defining permitted uses, auditing access, providing a reasonable opportunity to withdraw consent where possible, and reporting new uses to the public. Broad consent is not a blank check; it is acceptable only where trustworthy institutions limit what may be done. Local oversight should therefore be connected to a national picture: an anonymized event registry, shared lessons, and guidance for new uses of information. The mechanism should preserve independence without becoming a punitive system that encourages concealment. The aim is to identify an early pattern - for example, similar complaints about explanation, withdrawal, or database management - before it becomes a crisis.

Community participation does not replace individual consent. Community representatives can identify sensitivities, suggest appropriate language, and examine whether research will return benefits to the population bearing the risk. Approval by a leader, local committee, or patient organization, however, does not replace the consent of each participant. The community's role is to improve the conditions and credibility of research, not to hand over the bodies or data of its members.

Meaningful participation includes early discussion during planning, publication of results even when they are not positive, and an explanation of what will happen when funding ends. This helps prevent a situation in which a community serves as a convenient source of participants but does not benefit from the knowledge or treatment produced.

Biological Data After the Study Ends

A blood sample can be stored for years and used in studies that were unknown when it was collected. Broad consent may be justified, but it must explain limits, security, commercial sharing, and the possibility of withdrawing consent insofar as possible. Identified, coded, and anonymized data should be distinguished. A promise that everything is anonymous is not credible when datasets can be combined to re-identify individuals. The participant should know who manages the repository and who approves new uses. When research produces a profitable product, a benefit-sharing question arises. Not every participant is entitled to a share of the profits, but the community should not bear risk and remain without access to the outcome. Arrangements may include post-trial care, local training, affordable pricing, or investment in services. The commitment should be established in advance rather than after the product succeeds. In this way, research justice becomes a condition of planning rather than a later gesture.

Protecting whistleblowers: research failures are sometimes first identified by a coordinator, nurse, or junior investigator. If hierarchy punishes doubt, the ethics committee receives only a partial picture. An institution should create a confidential reporting channel, protect against retaliation, and investigate complaints promptly. A policy on paper is not enough; employees need to know whom to contact and what will happen. High-quality internal reporting protects participants and the research itself. A culture that conceals a small deviation allows it to grow. After a safety event, participants should be updated when the information could affect their willingness to continue. Consent is an ongoing process, so new information requires reconsideration. The committee may require a protocol change, suspension, or notification. The balance between maintaining blinding and the right to know should be reasoned. Trust in science is not built on the promise that errors never occur, but on how they are identified, disclosed, and corrected.

Vulnerable Groups and Injustice in Participant Selection

The principle of justice is not exhausted by the fact that every participant signed. Research can be unfair even when consent is valid if it imposes risk on a group that is unlikely to benefit from the results. One should ask why prisoners, soldiers, students, employees, or poor patients were selected. Sometimes the reason is scientific; sometimes they are simply available and dependent. The ethics committee should examine whether a less vulnerable population could be recruited and whether the offer made to the group exploits authority. When employees are asked to participate in research led by a department head, recruitment and consent should preferably be conducted by someone who does not influence their employment. Quiet refusal - simply not responding to an invitation - should also be accepted without repeated approaches and pressure. Excessive protection of pregnant women, older adults, or people with disabilities can exclude them from knowledge and lead to treatment based on a different population. The question is not whether to include or exclude them categorically, but how to adapt the study, reduce risk, and construct consent. Research that omits vulnerable groups may harm them in the future; research that includes them without protection harms them in the present. The decision requires a specific justification rather than use of a general label.

Compensation, treatment after harm, and access to results: a participant who is harmed should not have to fight to prove that the injury is related to the study before receiving care. The mechanism for compensation and treatment should already be clear in the consent document: who pays, where to turn, and what is not conditional on waiving legal rights. Insurance coverage that no one knows how to activate is not protection. Institutions can publish anonymized data about injuries and response times, thereby showing that responsibility continues beyond data collection. Compensation is not an automatic admission of negligence; it recognizes that research asks a person to bear risk for public knowledge. The results of the study also belong, in a moral sense, to the participants. It is not necessary to provide every technical analysis, but a comprehensible summary should be supplied, including notice when the study is terminated or shows no benefit. Negative results matter because they prevent repeated studies and unnecessary risk. When the sponsor controls publication, a rule established in advance should protect investigators' independence. A participant who devoted time and body to research is entitled to know what was learned, rather than discover that the study disappeared because the result was not commercially attractive.

Dynamic Consent in Data Repositories

In a long-term repository, different levels of consent can be offered: use for a specific disease, broad medical research, recontact, or prohibition on commercial use. A digital interface can permit changes, but there must also be an alternative for people who are not connected. Complete deletion should not be promised where data have already been incorporated into research or anonymized; the limitation should be explained honestly. A trustworthy system sends updates about new categories of use and allows objection where possible. Consent then becomes not an event forgotten in an archive, but a continuing relationship with the repository. Artificial intelligence adds questions of bias and responsibility. A large dataset is not necessarily representative, and an algorithm may perform less well for a group that was underrepresented. An ethics committee should examine not only privacy but also outcomes: who is included, who is harmed by an error, and how a person can challenge a decision assisted by a model. When a commercial company receives access, ownership, profit, and secondary use should be defined. The public may consent to medical research but not to targeted advertising or premium-setting. That distinction should appear in data governance rather than remain a statement of intent.

Experimental Treatment When No Available Alternative Exists

A person with advanced disease is invited to a study after exhausting accepted treatment. Hope is high, so the investigator explains that the primary purpose is to assess safety and that benefit is uncertain. Supportive care that does not depend on participation is also presented, and another conversation is offered with a physician outside the research team. A day later, the participant explains in their own words that the study may not benefit them and that they may withdraw. Only then is consent obtained. The scenario does not eliminate hope; it prevents hope from becoming coercion. When no curative alternative exists, the very availability of a study creates power. Separating supportive care from participation, allowing time to think, and checking understanding help balance it. The ethics committee should examine not only the form but the actual recruitment conditions. The level of risk, identifiability, and the implications of use determine the depth of protection. A waiver of consent in certain circumstances is not a waiver of responsibility: information must be minimized, oversight maintained, and public transparency enabled. Precise distinctions avoid a situation in which every study is wrapped in the same form, while also avoiding the assumption that data are ownerless material.

The quality of research protection is also tested after the article is published. A pathway should remain available for reporting late harm, communicating a relevant finding, and providing access to results in understandable language. Publishing a negative result matters because it prevents repetition of risk and respects the contribution of participants. An institution should know which commitments continue beyond the grant and ensure that they are funded. Research responsibility does not end when the database is closed, but when knowledge and lessons have been returned to those who bore the burden. The final test of ethical research is not the number of approvals but the status of the participant throughout the process. Did the person know they could refuse? Did they understand that the purpose of research differs from individualized treatment? Was there someone to protect them in case of harm? Were the results published even when they disappointed the sponsor? Codes, committees, and forms are tools; they do not replace a culture in which it is permissible to stop, report, and change direction. The pursuit of knowledge becomes ethical when it recognizes that the person is not a means to the result but a partner whose rights limit the route to it.

A further practical test arises in genetic research where samples collected for a defined purpose are transferred to a commercial partner in another country. The participant previously signed broad research consent, but international transfer, commercial profit, and the possibility that incidental findings might be returned were not explained. The committee does not rely on the old wording; it re-examines the basis of consent, requires clear notification, and defines what will happen to those who do not respond. In this way, technological change does not become retroactive unlimited authorization.

Decentralized Research and Sensors in the Home

Clinical trials are gradually moving from the clinic into the home: applications, smart watches, delivery of medicines, and video calls make it possible to participate without attending a medical center. Accessibility may improve, but the boundaries of the study become less clear. Participants may not know when a device is collecting data, who can see them, or what happens when an alert is generated at a time when no team is available.

A decentralized protocol must define technical support, an alternative pathway for people who do not have an appropriate device, responsibility for responding to abnormal findings, and the possibility of stopping data collection without withdrawing from all care. It should also examine who bears the cost of internet access, equipment, and time. Otherwise, the study shifts expenses and risks from the institution to the home and presents that transfer as convenience.

Use in the home also blurs the distinction between daily life and the research site. Information about sleep, location, or activity may expose family members who did not consent to participate. Minimizing data to what is necessary, encryption, and a separate explanation of continuous collection become part of meaningful consent.

Incidental findings and the duty to return information: genetic testing and broad imaging may reveal a finding that was not the purpose of the study. The investigator stands between two risks: retaining medically meaningful information in the repository, or disclosing an uncertain result that may trigger anxiety and unnecessary testing. Policy should therefore be determined in advance rather than after the finding appears.

A reliable and actionable finding should be distinguished from a research signal with no clear clinical meaning. Participants should know what kinds of results will be returned, who will verify them, and who will provide counseling. Graduated choices can also be offered: receive only life-threatening information, receive every actionable finding, or prefer not to receive certain information.

Returning a result does not end with notification. It requires a clinical pathway, protection of relatives, and the opportunity to ask how the information may affect insurance, employment, or privacy. This preserves the balance between the right to know and the right not to turn every biological possibility into a medical identity.

Trial Registration and Publication of Negative Results

A study that is not registered in advance makes it possible to change the question after the fact, select only a favorable result, and present a secondary analysis as though it were the original aim. Public registration before recruitment defines what will be measured, the primary outcome, and the planned number of participants. It does not guarantee good science, but it creates a point of comparison between the plan and the publication.

A negative or inconclusive result is valuable information. When it remains in a drawer, other researchers may repeat an unhelpful study, while participants have borne risk without producing usable knowledge. Institutions and sponsors should define a deadline for publication or deposit of a summary even if a journal does not accept the article. Protection of trade secrets may justify a limited delay, not indefinite concealment.

Participants should receive a clear summary of the research results once they are established. The summary is not a promise of personal benefit and does not replace medical advice, but it recognizes that the individual contributed time, body, and information. It should explain what was found, what cannot be concluded, and how further information can be obtained.

Institutional review should compare the registration, the report to the ethics committee, and the publication. A discrepancy may be justified if the protocol changed because of safety concerns or new information, but it should be documented. Research transparency thus protects not only scientific credibility but also the meaning of the consent given at the outset.

Stopping a Study in Time: Benefit, Harm, and Futility

Ethics approval at the beginning of a study does not determine that it may continue until the last participant. Accumulating information may reveal unexpected harm, clear benefit, or a low likelihood of reaching an answer. In such situations, stopping is part of protection, not a managerial failure. The problem is that early stopping can also distort results if driven by media pressure, commercial pressure, or chance fluctuation.

Studies involving significant risk require a monitoring body that receives interim data and is independent of the recruiting team. The protocol should define in advance which signals trigger review, who may see the results, and how blinding is preserved. A clear criterion protects against two errors: continuing a dangerous study because money has already been invested, and stopping prematurely after an unstable fluctuation.

When a study is stopped, responsibility toward participants continues. They should be told what is known, offered follow-up or alternative treatment, their treating physician should be updated, and it should be determined whether special disclosure is required for people exposed to risk. A general notice on a website is insufficient when the information may change personal treatment.

Stopping because of benefit also requires caution. An early result does not always justify immediate transition to routine care, and fair access for participants and the public should be ensured. Documenting the rationale and publishing the result protect trust and prevent an important institutional decision from remaining beyond review.

Chain of Protection in Human-Subjects Research

Stage	Typical Risk	Protective Mechanism	Required Documentation
Planning	Selecting a convenient but vulnerable group	Scientific justification and justice review	Rationale for selecting the population
Recruitment	Confusion between treatment and research	Independent explainer and time for consultation	Participant questions and alternatives provided
Conduct	Adverse events or pressure to remain	Immediate reporting and right to withdraw	Deviations, harms, and withdrawals
Completion	Lack of care or information after the study	Follow-up plan and access to results	Medical response and communication to participants
Future use	Expansion of uses of samples and data	Graduated consent and ability to change	Permissions, transfers, and deletion requests

Ethical governance is tested precisely when research succeeds, funding is available, and pressure to publish is high. A clear division of roles, a protected reporting channel, and oversight that does not end with the initial approval prevent a situation in which every actor assumes someone else is responsible. The participant remains a person with rights even after their data enter a repository.

Chapter Three: The Autonomy Revolution - From the Physician's Duty to the Patient's Right

Opening Dilemma

A young patient asks to stop a burdensome treatment, while her parents demand that it continue at any cost. The team may be tempted to see the family either as a source of support or as an obstacle, but it must begin by asking who holds the decision-making authority and whether the patient has decision-making capacity. A private conversation with the patient makes it possible to determine whether she is under pressure. The family can then be invited, with her consent, and the goals and limits of treatment can be explained. Mediation is not intended to achieve agreement at any cost. Sometimes the final decision will remain painful, but the family will understand that the team has not abandoned the patient and that her position has been heard. When a person lacks capacity, disagreement among family members can paralyze treatment.

The patient is not merely a body in need of healing; the patient is a person seeking to remain the author of his or her own life.

From the 1960s onward, rights movements, criticism of institutions, social change, and a new bioethics converged to transform the patient from a passive object into a partner with a voice.

1. Rights Movements and the Politics of the Body

The revolution in patients' rights formed part of a broader wave of struggles against unchecked authority - civil rights, feminism, disability rights, and criticism of psychiatric institutions. Historically, during the 1960s and 1970s, automatic trust in government, universities, the military, and medicine began to erode. Groups that had been pushed to the margins of public discussion demanded representation, information, and control over decisions concerning their bodies and their lives.

Within healthcare itself, hospitals began publishing bills of rights, establishing ethics committees, and developing complaint mechanisms. The change was uneven: at times a document was posted on the wall while the hierarchy remained unchanged. The struggle of women over childbirth, contraception, and abortion, for example, exposed the fact that a medical decision is not neutral. It incorporates assumptions about family, sexuality, risk, and social roles, and the patient must therefore have authority over the values that guide her decision.

Rights discourse can liberate, but it can also weaken solidarity if every encounter is described as a confrontation between claimants. A public healthcare system needs individual rights alongside responsibility for the fair distribution of resources. Israeli society went through similar processes, partly later and in a distinctly local form: a shift from state-centered collectivism toward a language of rights, judicial review, and service consumerism. These developments prepared the ground for the 1996 legislation.

Embedding rights requires patient participation in the design of services, not merely protection during the individual encounter. Quality committees, experience measures, and public councils should also give a voice to people who are neither organized nor powerful.

2. The Birth of Bioethics and the Balance Among Four Principles

Key source: Beauchamp & Childress, 2019.

Bioethics provided a shared language for discussing dilemmas: autonomy, beneficence, nonmaleficence, and justice, yet no principle operates alone. Advances in dialysis, transplantation, ventilation, genetics, and intensive care created decisions that could no longer be resolved through technical skill alone. Who should receive a scarce resource, when treatment may be stopped, and what constitutes death became public questions.

At the institutional level, clinical ethics committees were intended to enable multidisciplinary discussion rather than a purely legal one. They bring together physicians, nurses, lawyers, clergy, and public representatives, but their value depends on accessibility and on avoiding their use as a tool to justify a decision that has already been made. A patient who requests treatment that has no medical benefit places autonomy in tension with nonmaleficence and justice. The right to choose is not necessarily a right to demand every intervention; conversely, the definition of "futility" must be transparent and must not conceal considerations of age, disability, or cost.

The issue is more complex still: the four principles are not a mathematical formula. They require interpretation within a social and cultural context. Excessive emphasis on autonomy may ignore dependence; excessive emphasis on beneficence may reintroduce paternalism. In Israel, the Patients' Rights Law emphasizes dignity, privacy, information, and consent, but it operates alongside the National Health Insurance Law and questions concerning the benefits basket. The encounter between the two laws is the encounter between autonomy and distributive justice.

Ethics training should work with real cases, identify competing values, and clarify who has authority to decide. A list of principles without practice may remain a slogan that offers little help at two in the morning on a crowded ward.

3. Information, Understanding, and Shared Decision-Making

The real transition from formal autonomy to meaningful autonomy occurs when medical information becomes a dialogue adapted to the person's values and ability to understand. Historically, the law initially focused on what the physician had a duty to disclose. It later became clear that a list of risks does not guarantee understanding. Models of shared decision-making sought to connect medical evidence with personal preferences.

Within the service system, decision aids, interpreters, visit summaries, and digital systems can reduce disparities. Yet short appointment times, professional jargon, and assumptions of prior knowledge disproportionately harm people with low health literacy. Two patients with the same diagnosis, for example, may choose differently: one may prefer aggressive treatment despite substantial side effects, while the other gives greater weight to quality of life. There is no single "medically correct" choice that can be derived from the data alone.

At the same time, the wish not to know can itself be an expression of autonomy. A person may ask for information to be given to a family member or ask the physician to make a direct recommendation. The duty is to determine the patient's preferred decision-making style, not to impose an individualistic model. In Israel, a multilingual and multicultural society, informed consent requires adaptation to Arabic, Russian, Amharic, and other languages, as well as sensitivity to the role of the family without erasing the person receiving treatment.

Understanding should be assessed through teach-back, information should be provided in stages, and time for reflection should be allowed when there is no urgency. Systems should reward the quality of communication, not only the number of procedures and the speed of discharge.

4. Privacy, Confidentiality, and Control of Information in the Digital Age

The right to privacy has evolved from a duty to remain silent about a secret heard in the room into a broader question of control over information flowing among organizations, databases, applications, and artificial-intelligence systems. Historically, the medical record was created as a professional tool for the caregiver and the institution. Over time, the patient's right to inspect the record, correct errors, and understand who has accessed the information came to be recognized. Digitalization expanded both accessibility and risk at the same time.

In practice, an information system can prevent duplication, improve continuity, and save lives. It can also enable access on an enormous scale, linkage of data, and secondary use for research, planning, or commerce. Authorization mechanisms and access logs have therefore become part of patients' rights. Genetic information concerns not only the individual but also relatives. Disclosure may support prevention but can affect insurance, employment, and family relationships. Consent should therefore address not only the test itself but also storage, sharing, and future use.

Absolute privacy may impair treatment and public health, yet "system needs" can easily become a magic phrase. Every use should satisfy a defined purpose, proportionality, security, and transparency. In Israel, Sections 18-20 of the Patients' Rights Law regulate information, confidentiality, and disclosure. The shift toward national records and predictive technologies requires interpreting these arrangements in the spirit of Basic Law: Human Dignity and Liberty and privacy law (Basic Law: Human Dignity and Liberty, 5752-1992).

Information governance is required: mapping uses, explaining them to the public, auditing algorithms, allowing challenges to automated decisions, and imposing sanctions for unauthorized access. Digital trust is a condition of care, not a technological luxury.

5. From the Right to Refuse to the Right to Fair Treatment

Autonomy includes the right to refuse, but patients' rights are not exhausted by negative liberty. They also require accessibility, equality, and quality - conditions without which choice is empty. Liberal law tended to begin with protection against coercion. The right-to-health movement broadened the view toward state duties to provide services and social conditions that make health possible.

From an institutional perspective, a patient may decline surgery, but choice has little meaning if the alternative is not funded, the wait is too long, or the service is inaccessible because of disability. This is the distinction between rights in the clinical encounter and the social right to health. A person who refuses a blood transfusion for religious reasons, for example, sharpens the boundary of professional authority. When that person has capacity and understands the consequences, respect for the person's wishes may prevail even over the team's desire to save life. With a minor or a person lacking capacity, the balance changes.

The right to health, however, is a right to the highest attainable standard, not a guarantee of perfect health or of every treatment. It is constrained by resources but imposes immediate duties of nondiscrimination, transparency, and a core level of services. In Israel, the connection between the Patients' Rights Law and the National Health Insurance Law creates a dual framework: respectful treatment and consent on one side, and a benefits basket together with principles of justice, equality, and mutual assistance on the other (CESCR, 2000).

A rights policy should combine freedom from coercion, the right to refuse, access to information, and a right to complain with investment in waiting times, workforce, peripheral regions, and accessibility. Otherwise, the law protects a person's dignity while that person waits for a service that never arrives.

Decision Framework: Partnership in Conditions of Dependence and Uncertainty

Shared decision-making is a planned process: presenting comparable options, clarifying values, adapting support, and setting a point at which the choice will be reviewed. This section focuses on tools that allow a person to decide even when ill, anxious, dependent on family, or required to choose among alternatives none of which is perfect.

Choice is not the delivery of a menu. What the developments described above shared was a challenge to institutions that spoke on behalf of the person without listening. In the treatment room, the change took the form of rights to information, privacy, consent, and refusal. Yet adopting a new language did not eliminate power differences. The physician still holds knowledge, terminology, and access to resources. Autonomy therefore does not require the physician simply to say, "You decide"; it requires the physician to turn complex knowledge into an explanation the patient can use and to state which option is recommended and why. A decision that respects a patient's wishes may increase risk; a decision intended to prevent harm may ignore a value the patient sees as central. Good reasoning makes the conflict visible rather than hiding it behind authority. It examines the seriousness of the risk, reversibility, alternatives, and the person's ability to understand. When uncertainty is substantial, it should be stated explicitly rather than presenting a statistical estimate as though it were a certain personal prediction. Informed consent is a process in which the person understands the purpose of treatment, expected benefit, material risks, alternatives, and the option of no treatment. The scope of explanation varies with the decision: there is no need to turn a routine procedure into a legal ceremony, but a risky or irreversible treatment requires time, room for questions, and sometimes a second conversation. The quality of consent is also measured by the quality of the explanation provided by the team.

Capacity Is Decision-Specific, Not a Label

Decision-making capacity is not determined by diagnosis alone. A person with mental illness, mild dementia, or an intellectual disability may understand a particular decision, especially when information is presented in an adapted way. Assessment should examine the ability to understand, appreciate personal significance, weigh options, and communicate a choice. Capacity also varies over time: pain, sedating medication, delirium, or anxiety may temporarily impair it. Instead of rushing to appoint a substitute decision-maker, support should first be attempted - plain language, communication aids, a break, a person chosen by the patient, or delay when safe. Some patients explicitly ask to make decisions together with family members; others prefer privacy. When the family asks that a serious diagnosis be concealed, the team should understand the concern but ask the patient how information should be received. It should not be assumed in advance that the patient prefers not to know. Equally, a family that the patient sees as part of identity and of the ability to choose should not be excluded. An online portal, a detailed form, or a professional leaflet may be technically available but practically inaccessible. A person who does not speak Hebrew, has difficulty reading, or lacks a smartphone depends on intermediaries. Professional interpretation is especially necessary in complex decisions; using a child or family member may filter information and undermine privacy. Genuine accessibility is not an optional service enhancement but a condition for consent to be valid and equal across groups.

Autonomy in a World of Information and Family

Digital privacy cannot be reduced to a slogan. Medical information moves among health funds, hospitals, laboratories, applications, and technology companies. The patient should know when an external tool is processing personal data and what choices are available. A general authorization that no one understands is not control over information. One person's result may point to a preventable risk in others. Confidentiality remains the starting point, but the team should discuss safe ways of sharing with the patient, offer support, and assess the severity of the risk and the possibility of prevention. A departure from confidentiality, if the law permits it in extreme circumstances, should be narrow and a last resort. Advance directives and powers of attorney seek to protect the person's wishes when capacity is lost. Their interpretation should therefore also rely on values, earlier conversations, and familiarity with the person.

A proxy is not asked what the proxy personally would want, but what the person would have chosen or what is consistent with that person's welfare and values. Early conversations with family and the care team are as important as the signature because they reduce disagreement when the difficult moment arrives. Medical artificial intelligence adds a new layer of authority. A system may recommend a test, risk score, or treatment pathway, but the recommendation is not exempt from explanation simply because it rests on large quantities of data. The patient is entitled to know that such a tool influenced the decision, and the team must be able to assess whether the recommendation fits the individual before them. An algorithm trained on a different population may introduce bias; an interface that presents a single definitive score may crowd out judgment. Responsibility remains with the institution and the professionals, not with the software.

How shared decision-making can be evaluated: one can examine whether patients were able to describe the options, whether a recommendation was presented, whether an opportunity to ask questions was provided, and whether people who had difficulty received appropriate adjustments. In complex records, it is possible to examine whether the person's goals were documented rather than only the risks disclosed. Complaints about pressure, contradictory information, or family involvement against the patient's wishes should also become learning material. A good measure does not penalize the existence of disagreement; it asks whether the disagreement was managed respectfully and transparently. Professional training should include practice in real conversations: refusal of treatment, a family request to conceal information, uncertainty, and decisions in which there is no perfect option. Feedback should address not only medical accuracy but also pace, language, and the ability to recognize silence or agreement born of fear. Teams need adequate time and space; shared decision-making cannot be demanded while appointments are designed in a way that leaves no room for conversation. Working conditions are part of ethics because they determine whether the principle can be realized or remains a slogan.

Decision Fatigue in Chronic Illness

In chronic illness, autonomy is sometimes eroded not by one major decision but by dozens of small choices: dosage, nutrition, tests, appointments, and workplace adjustments. This burden creates decision fatigue and may appear to the team as nonadherence. Instead of adding more instructions, the patient and team should jointly define a limited set of priorities, choose one or two goals, and return to them at a fixed time.

A good plan includes the option to change direction. A preference chosen at the beginning of an illness is not a lifelong commitment; side effects, family circumstances, or changing values may justify reconsideration. Documenting the review point prevents an old decision from continuing merely through inertia.

Children, Adolescents, and the Transition to Adulthood

Parents make decisions for children, but the child is entitled to an age-appropriate explanation and to increasing participation. Parental consent does not eliminate the need to hear fear, pain, and resistance. Adolescents should have room for privacy, especially in sensitive matters, in accordance with law and circumstances. The team should explain to parents that partial privacy can improve trust and safety. When danger is present, the boundaries change, but the exception should be explained as far as possible. The transition from pediatric to adult medicine is a point of risk. A young person with chronic illness may lose a familiar team and a system in which parents managed everything. Preparation should begin early: learning medications, scheduling appointments, understanding rights, and developing the ability to ask questions independently. Parents move from managers to supporters. A gradual process prevents the young person from falling between frameworks and enables the development of real autonomy rather than imposing sudden independence on a particular birthday.

Mental Health and the Right to a Voice Even in Crisis

A mental-health crisis can impair judgment but does not automatically erase every preference. Capacity should be examined in relation to the specific decision, advance directives should be used, and the less restrictive intervention should be preferred. A person can explain in advance what is calming, who should be contacted, and which treatments have previously been experienced as harmful. A jointly prepared crisis plan allows the team to act quickly without starting from zero. When coercion is required, it should be reviewed frequently and participation should resume as soon as possible. After the crisis, a debriefing conversation is important. The patient receives an explanation of what was done, the team hears what was experienced as threatening, and both sides identify a different approach for the future. The conversation does not negate the need for treatment or limits, but it restores agency. It may also expose errors in communication or environment. Autonomy is not only the ability to say yes or no; it is the ability to influence how a person will be treated when that person's voice is weakened.

When There Is No Good Option - A Conversation About Uncertainty

Some medical decisions are not choices between good and bad treatment but between different risks. In such situations, the team may hide behind percentages or present a recommendation as if it were certain. A professional conversation should distinguish what is known at the group level from what can be predicted for the individual. Absolute numbers, ranges, and scenarios can be used instead of vague expressions such as "small risk." The person should be asked which kind of uncertainty is harder to bear: the risk of disease, the side effects, or the possibility of regret. Acknowledging that there is no perfect answer does not weaken the physician; it enables an honest decision. When the patient says to the physician, "Decide for me," this should not be interpreted as a surrender of rights. Sometimes the patient is asking for a strong recommendation because of trust or emotional overload. The physician can say what he or she would recommend and why, and clarify which values guided that recommendation. It is also worth asking whether the person wants the physician to make the decision or merely to help narrow the options. Voluntarily delegating a decision is different from having a decision taken away. Brief documentation of the preference and the reasons protects both sides and allows the issue to be revisited if circumstances change.

Supporting a decision without replacing the person's will: when the patient has difficulty expressing himself or herself, the family may provide essential context, but its role should be to support the decision rather than take its place. The team can clarify whom the patient wishes to involve, what values have guided the person in the past, and what the patient is currently able to understand and express. Support may include interpretation, visual aids, additional time, or breaking the decision into stages.

If the family seeks an outcome that contradicts the patient's wishes, the discussion should return to the question of who will bear the consequences of the decision. In a continuing dispute, an ethics or professional consultant who is not aligned with either side can be involved, while preserving the therapeutic relationship rather than resorting to a forceful ruling.

Concluding Case: The Same Medical Benefit, Different Priorities

Two treatments offer similar chances of survival. The first requires frequent visits and substantial side effects but allows close monitoring; the second is more convenient in daily life but involves greater uncertainty. The question is not which treatment is abstractly "better," but what price each person is willing to pay for stability, independence, or a sense of security.

The physician presents both options using the same measures, checks understanding, and asks the patient to describe a typical day under each pathway. The exercise reveals preferences that do not always emerge from a general question. After the choice, a date for reassessment is set, because actual experience may change the weight given to each advantage and disadvantage.

The case demonstrates that shared decision-making is not a compromise between the physician's opinion and the patient's wishes. It is the construction of a professional recommendation that takes account of medical information and of the life into which the decision will enter.

A patient with hearing loss arrives with her daughter to discuss surgery. The daughter answers every question quickly, and the physician assumes that this makes things easier for the mother. Only after an amplification device is used and the physician speaks directly with the patient does it become clear that the patient prefers conservative treatment, while the daughter is worried about the burden of care at home. Shared decision-making here requires two separate inquiries: what does the patient want, and what support is the family missing? A home-based service solution may change the choice without turning the daughter's voice into a substitute for the mother's.

Numeracy and Risk Communication

Many patients understand words but struggle to interpret probability. A statement that a treatment reduces risk by fifty percent may describe a reduction from two cases to one per thousand, or from fifty to twenty-five per hundred. Without the baseline risk, the impressive figure does not support an informed choice. Risk should therefore be presented in absolute terms, using the same time horizon and the same unit of measurement for each alternative.

A simple visual display can help, but it too may mislead if color, size, or the order of options emphasizes one outcome. It is preferable to use the same symbols, show both benefit and harm, and check understanding by asking the patient to explain the information in his or her own words. The purpose is not to test the patient but to discover where misunderstanding lies.

When the data are uncertain, that uncertainty should be stated explicitly. The range, quality of evidence, and difference between a group average and an individual outcome are as important as the number itself. Good risk communication allows a person to decide even in the absence of guarantees, without turning uncertainty into concealment or intimidation.

Digital Decision Aids and Hidden Bias

A digital system can organize options, ask about preferences, and produce a summary for discussion. It may expand participation, but the order of questions, default settings, and the way risk is displayed influence the result. A tool funded by a manufacturer or designed to reduce costs may subtly steer the user toward a particular choice without the patient realizing it.

Disclosure of information sources and funding is therefore necessary, along with accessibility testing across different groups and the ability to see how a recommendation was generated. The aid does not replace a conversation, especially when the decision is emotionally charged or when the person has difficulty reading. Its role is to prepare for the conversation and document preferences, not to turn an algorithmic recommendation into consent.

Advance Directives as a Bridge Across Time

A relatively healthy person may find it difficult to imagine how he or she will feel in a state of serious illness, so an advance directive is not a perfect forecast. Its value lies in creating a conversation about values: what matters more - prolonging life, the ability to communicate, independence, or avoiding suffering? These values can also guide decisions when the exact scenario was not written into the document.

Directives should be updated after a new diagnosis or a change in family circumstances, and the team should ensure that they are available in real time. A document kept in a drawer does not protect autonomy. Incorporating it into the medical record, appointing a person who knows the patient's wishes, and repeating the conversation turn it into a living tool.

The right not to decide immediately: autonomy discourse tends to assume that presenting information should end in an immediate choice. In practice, a decision may be better precisely because the person asks for time. A new diagnosis, fatigue, pain, or emotional overload can impair the ability to connect information with one's life. As long as a short delay does not create unreasonable risk, a request to think, consult, or return to the conversation is part of consent and not a sign of noncooperation.

The team should distinguish medical urgency from organizational urgency. An operating schedule, physician rounds, or the desire to complete a discharge does not make a decision impossible to postpone. When time truly is limited, the team should explain what will happen if the decision is delayed, which part must be done now, and which choices can remain for later. Breaking the decision into parts prevents fear of losing a treatment window from becoming pressure to accept an entire package.

Sometimes it is possible to offer a reversible, time-limited treatment trial. Instead of demanding a long-term commitment, the team defines a goal, duration, stopping criteria, and a date for reassessment. This model is particularly appropriate when benefit is uncertain and the burden depends on personal experience. It does not postpone the decision forever; it turns uncertainty into part of a plan that can be tested.

Documentation of a delay should show that the person was given a route back into the system, not merely that the person "refused." It should state who will make contact, what additional information will be provided, and which warning signs require earlier consultation. In this way, the right to time does not become abandonment, and professional responsibility continues even while the decision remains open.

Adapting the Decision Process to the Person's Situation

The quality of autonomy is not measured by the number of options presented, but by the extent to which the person was able to connect those options to his or her life. A good decision may include a clear medical recommendation and help from family, as long as there remains room for questions, an option to change course, and a distinction between support and takeover.

Decision Situation	Main Barrier	Required Adaptation	Desired Outcome
Choosing between treatments	Information overload and anxiety	Comparison using the same measures and clarification of priorities	A choice the person can explain
Chronic illness	Changing circumstances over time	Review points and an adaptable plan	Adherence that is not based on coercion

Decision Situation	**Main Barrier**	**Required Adaptation**	**Desired Outcome**
Temporary cognitive difficulty	Pain, medication, or fatigue	A break, assistive tools, and repeated explanation	Decision-specific assessment rather than a global label
Family involvement	The relative's voice takes over	Clarification of who has authority and what the patient requested	Partnership that does not erase the individual
High uncertainty	A recommendation presented as certainty	Presentation of the limits of knowledge and an alternative plan	Ability to change direction without a sense of failure

Part Two: The State of Israel - From Paternalistic Hegemony to Advanced Legislation

The Israeli story is not a copy of the American or European development. It emerged from the medicine of the Yishuv, the health funds, mass immigration, the military, public hospitals, and an ethos of nation-building. These institutions rapidly expanded access to care and produced impressive achievements, but they also fostered a culture in which the profession and the system sometimes presumed to know better than the individual. Part Two examines how this balance changed and how it matured into the Patients' Rights Law.

Chapter Four: The Era of Institutional Medicine - From the 1950s to the 1980s

Opening Dilemma

An older woman who does not speak Hebrew arrives with her son for an appointment at which an oncologic diagnosis is disclosed. The son asks the physician "not to tell her everything" in order to preserve her hope. The physician speaks mainly to him, and the woman understands that the matter is serious but does not know what has been decided. The professional response is neither to ignore the family nor immediately disclose information contrary to the patient's possible wishes. With the help of an interpreter, the team should ask her how she prefers to receive information and whom she wants involved. Only she can determine whether the son is a supporter, a representative, or someone who should not hear certain details.

The state sought to heal a public; the individual sought not to disappear within that public.

Early Israeli medicine was built on solidarity, mission, and strong institutions; paradoxically, its public success contributed to a situation in which the patient's voice remained secondary for many years to professional authority and collective needs.

1. Health as Nation-Building

In the first years of statehood, health was viewed as part of a national mission of absorbing immigrants, preventing epidemics, training personnel, and rebuilding society after war and mass migration. Historically, the young state faced immigrant camps, transit camps, infectious diseases, shortages of beds and staff, and major disparities between the center and the periphery. The health funds, the Ministry of Health, Hadassah, and other institutions operated in a reality of constant urgency.

At the institutional level, such conditions favored uniformity, vaccination, rapid triage, and population-level solutions. The public logic was understandable: when resources are limited and risk is collective, it is difficult to organize every treatment around individual preferences. Mass public-health campaigns illustrate the tension. They can save many lives and reduce inequality, but when they are conducted without explanation, cultural adaptation, or the possibility of asking questions, they can leave a memory of coercion even when the intention was beneficial.

At the same time, anachronistic judgment should be avoided. The concepts and resources of patients' rights were not developed as they are today. Yet recognizing historical circumstances does not require silencing the testimonies of people who experienced humiliation, concealment of information, or discriminatory treatment. In Israel, the state-building ethos connected medicine with citizenship, work, and security. It expanded services but also created an expectation of compliance. "Trust the doctor" expressed both confidence and dependence.

The lesson is that emergency and public policy do not exempt institutions from transparency. Even in a broad campaign, purpose, risk, and alternatives should be explained, community leadership should be involved, and documentation should be preserved so that retrospective review is possible.

2. The Health Funds and Community Medicine

The health funds created a distinctive Israeli tradition of organizational responsibility and community medicine, but membership in a health fund did not necessarily give the patient a defined and transparent bundle of enforceable rights. Historically, even before statehood, health funds operated within labor movements and public organizations. Over the years they became the main gateway to healthcare, with clinics, family physicians, pharmacies, and hospitals.

When translated into practice, the health fund combined financing with service provision. This integration enabled continuity and responsibility for a population, but it also created situations in which decisions about eligibility, referrals, and the covered basket were sometimes opaque, and patients had difficulty knowing what they were entitled to and what could be appealed. A refusal to refer a patient for an expensive test, for example, may reflect a medical judgment, a budgetary judgment, or a combination of both. Without reasons and an appeal pathway, the patient does not know which authority is being exercised.

Resource management is nevertheless unavoidable. A public system cannot promise every service to every person, but it must distinguish among professional judgment, organizational constraint, and budgetary decision-making, and present the distinction in a way that can be understood and reviewed. As the 1990s approached, Israel moved toward a more explicit public framework, which will be discussed in the next chapter. The importance of that shift here lies in what preceded it: a patient who did not always know the scope of entitlement, who had set it, or what could be appealed.

A practical right requires a clear written decision, published procedures, exceptions committees, timelines for appeals, and assistance for patients who cannot navigate the system on their own. Transparency is a component of equality.

3. The Israeli Hospital and the Hierarchy of Knowledge

The Israeli hospital developed as a powerful professional institution in which respect for authority, workload, and bedside training tended to push personal conversation to the margins. The expansion of hospitals, introduction of advanced technologies, and development of specialist professions created centers of excellence. At the same time, a clear hierarchy remained among department directors, senior physicians, residents, nurses, and allied health professionals.

From an applied perspective, hierarchy enables rapid decisions and professional supervision, but it can silence both junior staff and patients. When a staff member is afraid to challenge a senior physician, it is difficult to expect a patient to do so. Morning rounds are a moment in which critical decisions are made. If the discussion takes place over the patient's head in professional language, the patient is physically present but absent from the process that determines his or her life.

A crowded ward cannot be run as a permanent assembly. It is nevertheless possible to distinguish professional discussion from the conversation with the patient, present conclusions in understandable language, and ensure an opportunity for questions. In Israel, an organizational culture of improvisation, speed, and "it will be all right" sometimes contributed to impressive flexibility and sometimes to weak documentation. The Patients' Rights Law imposed an explicit requirement for a medical record, information, and consent.

Change requires departmental leadership, communication rules, protected time for explanation, and empowerment of nurses and other professions as partners in safeguarding rights. Safety and dignity depend on the ability of every person in the room to speak.

4. Immigration, Culture, and Inequality

The healthcare system served as a central instrument of immigrant absorption, but encounters between professional knowledge and different groups exposed disparities of language, status, race, and culture that affected the ability to exercise rights. Historically, waves of immigration from different countries brought varied understandings of the body, family, authority, and illness. The system had to act quickly and at times interpreted cultural difference as lack of understanding or irrational resistance.

Organizationally, professional interpreting was almost entirely absent from routine services for many years. Family members, and sometimes children, translated sensitive information. This harmed confidentiality, accuracy, and freedom to refuse. When a woman depends on her partner for translation, for example, there is no way to know whether she receives all the information or whether her wishes are heard. Family interpretation may be convenient for the system but may alter the decision itself.

Cultural sensitivity does not mean uncritical acceptance of every practice. The system must protect people from violence and coercion, but it should do so through listening and understanding rather than stereotype. In Israel, disparities between Jews and Arabs, center and periphery, immigrants and long-established residents, and religious and secular groups are not merely epidemiological data; they affect information, trust, waiting times, and the ability to challenge decisions.

Structured interpreting services, accessible documents, a diverse workforce, measurement of disparities, and community participation are required. Nondiscrimination is not merely a prohibition on hostile treatment; it is an obligation to design a service that can actually be used.

5. The Absence of a Unified Legal Framework and Reliance on Ethics and Case Law

Until the 1990s, patients' rights in Israel rested on scattered rules, tort law, professional ethics, and case law; protection existed but was partial, inaccessible, and inconsistent. Historically, professional ordinances, confidentiality rules, and the law of assault and negligence provided some framework. Courts dealt with consent and duties of disclosure, but there was no single charter explaining to patients and institutions the full set of rights.

In practice, this fragmentation created dependence on legal knowledge and on the ability to sue after harm had already occurred. It provided almost no preventive tools for care teams or simple mechanism for resolving disputes in real time. A patient who wanted to inspect the record or receive an explanation had to rely on an internal procedure, goodwill, or a lawyer. The right was not always visible even if it could be inferred from general principles.

Reality, however, is more complex: uniform legislation can harden discretion and encourage defensive medicine. On the other hand, the absence of law leaves the boundary in the hands of the stronger institution. The challenge is to establish a clear core while allowing flexibility in implementation. In Israel, the 1996 law was intended to turn familiar values into defined duties: proper medical treatment, nondiscrimination, information, consent, confidentiality, and a medical record. It did not create every principle from nothing, but consolidated, strengthened, and made them more accessible.

Even after legislation, professional codes and case law remain necessary. The law provides a floor; ethics can set a higher standard, and judicial decisions interpret situations that cannot be anticipated in advance.

Institutional Review: The Nation-Building Legacy and the Cost of Uniformity

The Israeli system was built under conditions of urgency, mass migration, and scarcity. This section examines how patterns born in that period - uniformity, discipline, centralization, and reliance on mission - continue to influence language, peripheral regions, patient representation, and the ability to adapt services without abandoning a common public floor.

Public Medicine Under Conditions of National Emergency

Epidemic prevention, vaccination, hospitalization, and the establishment of clinics often came before lengthy discussion of preferences. The context explains why a paternalistic culture developed, but it does not erase the price paid by those unfamiliar with the language and rules of the institution. A new immigrant could receive essential treatment while not understanding what was being done or why. Formal equality - the same clinic and the same procedure - did not guarantee an equal ability to use the service. Those who arrived with connections, Hebrew, or familiarity with the system could ask questions; others were expected to comply. Links to labor organizations and political frameworks provided infrastructure but also affected belonging and access. A clear hierarchy developed in hospitals: the senior physician made the decision, while the nurse sometimes knew the patient's fears, language, and ability to understand better than anyone else.

That knowledge did not always reach the decision table. The case illustrates that multidisciplinary teamwork is not merely an organizational improvement; it is a way of restoring information and presence to the patient when both have disappeared inside hierarchy. Military and emergency medicine contributed values of mission, discipline, and speed. In disaster situations these values save lives. The problem begins when command language continues into routine care: a question is seen as an interruption, hesitation as noncooperation, and the family as an instrument for carrying out a decision already made. A mature system must know how to shift between modes. In a trauma room it is possible to act quickly and return to explanation after stabilization; in a chronic-care clinic there is no justification for reproducing the emergency pattern. Distinguishing true urgency from organizational urgency is a condition of rights.

Language Is More Than Translating Words: a language barrier is not limited to unfamiliarity with a medical term. Diagnosis, risk, confidentiality, and consent acquire meaning within culture, family relationships, and prior experience with government. Using a child as an interpreter may expose the child to age-inappropriate information, undermine privacy, and impose responsibility the child cannot bear. An adult family member can help, but may also filter information or speak in place of the patient. Professional interpretation is therefore part of patient safety. It is especially necessary for difficult decisions, intimate examinations, and situations in which consent or refusal depends on precise understanding. An effective interpretation service does not begin with a phone call to an interpreter. The institution should know in advance which languages are common, how services are obtained outside normal hours, and what to do when there is no immediate response.

The staff member should speak to the patient rather than to the interpreter, use short sentences, and pause to check understanding. The language used for explanation and the person's preference regarding family involvement should be documented, while sweeping labels such as "traditional family" should be avoided. Cultural adaptation means professional curiosity, not an assumption that every person from a particular group wants the same thing. The medical record also reflects power relations. For years it was written as an internal professional tool in language intended for colleagues. Once the patient gained a right to inspect it, the meaning of the words changed. A derogatory, judgmental, or vague description is not only a stylistic matter; it can influence future treatment and trust. The risk is particularly high in the path of a new immigrant, because an error in a name, family status, or understanding of history can move between institutions without the person knowing how to correct it. The right to inspect the record should be accompanied by a simple way to request correction and explanation in accessible language.

A Serious Diagnosis Through a Family Member: the scenario shows that Israeli autonomy does not have to be individualistic. When an institution assumes in advance that a family from a particular group decides for the patient, it replaces medical paternalism with cultural paternalism. Conversely, removing the family from the room in the name of independence may harm the patient's main source of support. The test is the person's wishes, not the image of the group to which that person belongs.

From the Past to Contemporary Policy: improving accessibility requires more than translating leaflets. It is necessary to map where the pathway breaks down: scheduling, reception, the clinical conversation, discharge, or complaint. A different role-holder is responsible at each point. The scheduling center should identify language needs; the ward should order an interpreter; the physician and nurse are responsible for checking understanding; management allocates resources; and the health fund or hospital must permit communication even for someone who cannot write in Hebrew. Such mapping replaces the assumption that the patient "did not cooperate" with a practical question: where was the person not given a real opportunity to understand? Appropriate measurement may include the rate of interpreter use in complex decisions, waiting time for the service, complaints about misunderstanding, medication errors after discharge, and disparities between language groups. The data do not tell the whole story. Conversations with patients and staff can show whether the service arrived in time and whether the interpreter was appropriate for the subject. Institutions should not be compared without considering population composition and quality of reporting. An institution that identifies more disparities is not necessarily worse; it may simply give people more room to speak.

The goal is to improve the pathway, not to punish the act of discovering problems. The gap between center and periphery accumulates through language, transportation, specialist availability, and the ability to miss work. A clinic that exists on the map is not accessible if there is no way to reach it or if every explanation is given in an unfamiliar language. Remote interpretation can be used in small sites, but it is not suitable for every conversation. Intimate examinations, cognitive impairment, or end-of-life discussion may require in-person presence. Local adaptation is not a lowering of standards, but selection of the means that realizes the standard. Nurses should be permanent partners in planning. They see patients over time, identify gaps in understanding after the physician leaves the room, and often deal with the consequences of instructions that were not understood. Giving a nurse authority to order an interpreter, briefly delay discharge to clarify a problem, or raise a concern does not undermine hierarchy; it is a safety mechanism. Administrative staff also matter: a right can fail even before the clinical encounter when a form, code, or scheduling system is inaccessible.

Immigrant Absorption Between Mission and Standardization

Professionals sometimes acted from a deep sense of mission, but institutional language tended to view immigrants as a population that needed to be educated and adapted. Medical explanation became intertwined with a cultural message about hygiene, family, and nutrition. The historical test is not only whether services were established, but whether people could understand, ask, and preserve their dignity. Camps and transit camps illustrated how living conditions determine health. An instruction to ventilate, isolate, or maintain a particular diet is impossible to follow when there is no space, water, or money. The contemporary lesson is that personal responsibility cannot be separated from conditions. A service that asks for behavioral change should ask what is required to make that change possible and who can provide the resource.

Military Medicine and Its Influence on the Civilian System

The military framework contributed organization, emergency readiness, and the capacity for rapid action. It also reinforced a culture of hierarchy, orders, and postponement of personal needs in favor of the mission. When that pattern moves into civilian care, it may help in disaster but harm ordinary conversation. A patient is not a soldier, and refusal is not necessarily a breach of discipline. Management training should distinguish emergency situations requiring decisive action from routine care in which time for explanation is part of treatment. At the same time, military service created training pathways and movement of knowledge between periphery and center. Professionals encountered different populations and developed improvisational skills. The history is complex: the same institution can expand access and strengthen paternalism. A balanced discussion does not search for one-dimensional blame, but identifies which characteristics should be preserved - responsibility, preparedness, and coordination - and which should be limited - obedience, institutional secrecy, and the assumption that the individual must adapt to the system.

Childbirth, Motherhood, and Women's Voices

Maternity institutions reduced mortality and provided care, but moved childbirth from the home into a space in which staff determined position, presence, and procedures. Women from different groups sometimes experienced judgmental treatment or little explanation. The right to consent in childbirth developed later, but historically it is possible to examine the ability to choose a companion, understand an intervention, and express pain. Personal testimonies are important because the medical record documents the clinical outcome but not always the experience. The tension between public health and autonomy is also visible in fertility policy. Encouragement of childbirth, prevention, or treatment can carry different meanings for different groups. To assess a policy, one should ask who formulated it, what information was provided, and which options were available. A national intention does not cancel the private body.

The Periphery as a Problem of Time, Continuity, and Professional Presence

Geographic distance is only one component of medical peripherality. An appointment that requires an entire workday, lack of transportation, high physician turnover, and transfer of a patient among centers create disparities even when a clinic appears on the map. Measuring accessibility should therefore include travel time, waiting time, number of changes of caregiver, and the ability to receive follow-up treatment along the same pathway.

The correction does not have to consist of fully replicating a large medical center. A stable team can be strengthened, remote consultation can be linked to local examination, coordinated transportation can be provided, and a referral pathway can accompany the person until the service is actually received. This preserves centralized expertise without turning the patient into the logistical manager of the system.

Immigration, Prevention, and the Power of the State: policies of screening, vaccination, and isolation are designed to protect a large public, but they operate with particular force on people who depend on the state for housing, work, and status. A person in a transit camp or absorption center may find it difficult to refuse even when there is no explicit coercion. Public health therefore requires explanation, a way to obtain information, and oversight of proportionality. When an action is required to protect others, that should be said openly rather than presented as an individual therapeutic decision. Distinguishing treatment for the person's benefit from action for the benefit of the public enables an honest discussion of the limits of power. The history of immigration also includes knowledge that went unrecognized. Institutions can learn from it without abandoning evidence. When a person uses an herb, traditional healer, or ritual, the first question is not whether that person "believes in science," but whether there is a dangerous interaction and what the practice means to the individual.

Curious conversation makes it possible to identify risk and build trust. Ridicule or blanket prohibition drives the practice outside the conversation and increases danger.

Representing the Patient Within the Team: nursing and the therapeutic professions can bridge the language of the system and the person's life, but only if their voices are heard. Team meetings can include not only diagnosis and results but also understanding, support at home, and social barriers. A nurse who realizes that the patient does not understand discharge instructions should be able to stop the process without fearing that this will be seen as obstructing throughput. A social worker should enter the process before an economic crisis develops. Multidisciplinary care is not simply many people around a bed; it is the integration of different types of knowledge into the decision. Public and community representatives should also be diverse. A recognized leader does not necessarily represent women, young people, people with disabilities, or people who are not organized. Consultation can take place in small groups, in different languages, and in places where people feel safe. Information collected should return to the public with an explanation of what was accepted and what was not. Otherwise participation becomes a ritual seeking legitimacy for a decision already made.

An Archive of Silences: What Can Be Learned from What Was Not Documented

Institutional documents usually record management decisions, budgets, and achievements, but almost never preserve the conversation in which a patient did not understand, the nurse who mediated between languages, or the family that had to improvise a solution. The history of patients' rights therefore cannot rely on official protocols alone. Letters, newspapers, oral testimony, court files, and training materials must also be included.

Silence itself is a finding. The absence of complaints does not prove satisfaction when there was no clear address for complaints, when the complainant depended on the same institution, or when legal language was inaccessible. Comparing what an institution reported with what appears in private testimony helps identify the gap between public mission and everyday experience.

Preserving the archives of health funds, hospitals, and immigrant organizations is therefore a policy tool and not merely an academic concern. It allows us to understand which patterns recur, which adaptations were lost when management changed, and how a legacy can be corrected without erasing its contribution.

Public Health, Vaccination, and the Limits of Coercion

The young State of Israel had to confront infectious diseases, overcrowding, and difficult living conditions. Vaccination, screening, and hygiene campaigns saved lives, but they sometimes relied on a language of discipline and on substantial power differences between the state and immigrants or disadvantaged populations. The tension between the public good and individual choice was not theoretical; it appeared in schools, transit camps, and clinics.

A justified public intervention requires a scientific basis, proportionality, and explanation. Where there is a less intrusive alternative - education, accessibility, reminders, or language adaptation - coercion should not be the first response. Even during an outbreak, it should be clear who has authority to order a measure, for how long, and how it can be challenged. Transparency about risk and side effects does not weaken a vaccination campaign; it prevents the sense that information is being held by those in power.

History shows that trust damaged during an emergency can influence behavior for years. Documentation, apology, and correction are therefore not merely symbolic. They are part of the state's future ability to ask the same community for cooperation.

Nurses and Social Workers as System Mediators

During periods of immigrant absorption and scarcity, community nurses and social workers sometimes knew the family better than the central institution did. They translated not only language but also patterns of daily life, fears, and the practical ability to reach treatment. This knowledge was essential but did not always receive status in decision-making or documentation.

A centralized system may see mediation as a departure from uniformity. In fact, good mediation makes it possible to preserve a professional standard while adapting the route. A home visit, transportation coordination, explanation to a family member, or change of appointment time is not an abandonment of equality; these are means of achieving a more equal outcome.

Recognizing these roles requires protected work time, training, and authority to raise problems. When mediation rests only on personal dedication, it disappears when the employee changes. Making it part of the system preserves knowledge and reduces dependence on chance.

Institutional Mental Health and the Voice Left Outside the Record

Psychiatric hospitals and mental-health services in the early decades operated within a culture that gave substantial weight to diagnosis, order, and protection. In situations of danger, a structured setting was genuinely necessary, but broad definitions of noncooperation sometimes allowed restrictions on movement, communication, and family contact without sufficient examination of wishes and capacity.

A psychiatric record tends to accompany a person for a long time and influence how teams interpret later behavior. A sentence written during a crisis can become a permanent explanation for every physical complaint or disagreement. The history of patients' rights should therefore include the right to be heard even during severe mental distress and the duty to distinguish among symptom, disagreement, and actual risk.

Correction does not mean abandoning safety. It requires a clear basis for restriction, repeated review, explanation as far as possible, and an external avenue of oversight. The presence of an advocate, family member, or staff member outside the coercive chain can balance power and bring forward information the ward does not see.

The historical perspective explains why people who experienced involuntary hospitalization or institutional labeling may fear even a modern system. Building trust begins by acknowledging the experience, separating the past from the present decision, and allowing inaccurate information to be corrected.

Mass-Casualty Triage and Equality Under Pressure

A system built through wars, waves of immigration, and emergencies developed the ability to triage rapidly and allocate resources. In a mass-casualty event, it is impossible to provide full treatment to everyone immediately, so the team prioritizes according to expected benefit, urgency, and available resources. The need for triage does not abolish rights; it changes the way the duty of fairness is realized.

A triage rule should be clinical, as transparent as possible, and revisable when circumstances change. Status, personal connections, language, or family pressure should not move someone ahead. A rapid label can persist even after a condition improves or worsens, so repeated reassessment is required rather than reliance on a label assigned at arrival.

Even under heavy workload, minimum information should be provided: the order of priority, who is monitoring the patient, and when another assessment will occur. A family that receives no explanation may interpret waiting as abandonment. A dedicated communication role allows the clinical team to work while reducing anxiety and conflict.

After the event, review should examine not only mortality and treatment time, but also who was transferred, who remained without information, and whether certain groups were consistently disadvantaged. Such a review connects Israel's emergency-care legacy with a modern language of equality, transparency, and learning.

Institutional Legacy: Asset, Cost, and Correction

Historical Pattern	**Contribution to the System**	**Possible Cost**	**Contemporary Correction**
Action in an emergency	Speed and organizational capacity	Reduced space for explanation	A procedure for moving from urgent action to a full conversation
Uniform service	A common public floor	Ignoring language and culture	Adaptations in the pathway, not only in the leaflet
Professional hierarchy	Clear decision-making and responsibility	Difficulty voicing disagreement	Patient representation and a team channel for stopping a process
Concentration of expertise	Quality in large centers	Time and travel costs for peripheral populations	Mobile services and regional coordination
The immigration-absorption mission	Rapid expansion of coverage	Labeling groups as a uniform population	Collecting preferences and community representation

History explains why patterns arose, but it does not grant them immunity. A system can preserve solidarity, emergency readiness, and strong public medicine while replacing blind uniformity with adaptation. Correction begins by identifying places where a procedure born of scarcity continues to operate even though a better alternative now exists.

Chapter Five: The Catalysts for Legislation - Public Criticism, Case Law, and Constitutional Revolution

Opening Dilemma

A family discovers after the fact that an invasive treatment was performed without a full explanation of a conservative alternative. The physician is convinced that the best option was chosen, and the treatment was medically successful. Before an explicit language of rights, the dispute might have ended with the statement that no harm was caused. Public criticism changes the question: were the patient and family given an opportunity to understand and decide? This does not imply that the physician acted maliciously; it recognizes that even benevolent expertise can deprive a person of a voice. From such a case arises the need for a rule that does not depend on the physician's personality or on the family's ability to create public controversy. At the same time, turning every conversation into a legal document may undermine the very purpose of the reform.

A law is not born on the day of the vote; it summarizes years of dissatisfaction, struggle, and change in language.

The Patients' Rights Law matured at the intersection of social change, developing case law, health legislation, public activism, and the rise of human dignity as a constitutional principle.

1. The Crisis of Trust and the Emergence of the Public Voice

As the public became more educated, more connected through media, and more mobile, the assumption that medical institutions were entitled to trust without explanation or criticism weakened. The expansion of the media, consumer organizations, patient groups, and the ability to compare treatments changed the balance of power. Errors and scandals that once remained inside institutions became matters of public concern.

At the system level, hospitals began appointing public-relations or complaints officers, publishing procedures, and recognizing that the service experience is part of quality. Yet a complaint was sometimes viewed as a threat to staff rather than as a source of learning. A family that receives no explanation after an adverse event, for example, may turn to the media or to court. The motive is not always compensation; sometimes the absence of information and apology is what escalates the dispute.

Transparency does not require an immediate determination of fault. Known facts can be shared, suffering can be acknowledged, and a review can be promised without compromising a professional investigation. Protective silence may be perceived as concealment. Israeli society is characterized by direct interaction and a willingness to challenge authority, yet the medical system retained a strong hierarchy for many years. The encounter between these two cultures created pressure for legislation.

An effective complaints system should be independent, accessible, and rapid, protect complainants against retaliation, and publish trends. The right to complain is part of care and not merely a stage on the way to litigation.

2. Case Law Before the Law and the Duty of Disclosure (CA 3108/91 Reibi; CA 4384/90 Vaturi)

Israeli courts gradually expanded the duty of disclosure and recognized that a medical decision includes a value-based choice belonging to the patient, not only the physician's professional judgment. Historically, medical-negligence decisions addressed information about risks, alternatives, and the scope of consent. The 1993 Reibi case is among the important milestones in the discussion that preceded the statute.

Within the service structure, case law operated retrospectively, after harm had occurred, but it influenced forms, documentation, and training. It turned clinical communication into a matter of legal responsibility, for better and for worse. When a treatment carries an uncommon risk with serious consequences, the question is not only whether a reasonable physician would mention it, but whether it is material to the decision of the particular patient.

A patient-based standard can make prediction difficult, while a purely professional standard can preserve concealment. A combination of medical practice, materiality of risk, and the patient's questions offers a more balanced framework. In Israel, the law adopted a broad list of required information: diagnosis, nature of treatment, expected benefit, risks, alternatives, and the risks of foregoing treatment. In doing so, it converted principles developed in case law into institutional guidance.

Training should teach not only "what must be said" but how to identify what matters to the person. Personalized documentation of the conversation is preferable to uniform text that does not reflect the real dilemma.

3. Basic Law: Human Dignity and Liberty and the Constitutional Change

The enactment of Basic Law: Human Dignity and Liberty in 1992 gave patients' rights discourse a constitutional anchor in dignity, liberty, privacy, and bodily integrity. Historically, the constitutional revolution did not explicitly create a right to health, but it changed legal thinking. Governmental and institutional actions were increasingly examined through fundamental rights and proportionality.

In clinical reality, human dignity concerns the way people are spoken to, bodily exposure, confidentiality, coercion, and recognition of the person as a subject. Liberty concerns consent and refusal; privacy concerns the body and information. Medical treatment without consent, for example, may save a life and still infringe dignity and liberty. Constitutional law does not provide an automatic answer, but it requires a proper purpose and proportionate means.

The absence of an explicit constitutional right to health leaves a gap between strong negative rights and claims for resources. It is easier to protect privacy than to compel the opening of a hospital department in a peripheral region. In Israel, the Patients' Rights Law, enacted four years after the Basic Law, uses the language of dignity and privacy and translates it into the clinical world. The two laws are read in light of one another.

Future interpretation should preserve the connection between dignity, quality, and accessibility. A person who receives courteous treatment but cannot obtain essential care does not enjoy a complete right.

4. Social Legislation, Rights Organizations, and Patient Groups

The legislation drew on the activity of members of Knesset, professionals, lawyers, rights organizations, and patient groups that turned private experiences into a public problem. A Patients' Rights Bill was published as early as 1992. The discussions continued for years and included disputes over consent, emergency treatment, ethics committees, confidentiality, and the right to die with dignity.

At the organizational level, civil-society organizations helped frame the issue not merely as service relations but as human rights. Patient groups contributed experiential knowledge, especially in psychiatry, disability, HIV, and chronic illness. The struggle over access to the medical record illustrates how an abstract right becomes a practical tool: it allows a person to understand treatment, obtain an opinion, correct an error, and restore a sense of control.

In concrete terms, the law should not be attributed to any single actor. Legislative processes are changing coalitions of interests, and organizations seeking broad protection sometimes accepted narrower compromises. In Israel, the Association for Civil Rights and other organizations continued their activity after enactment, for example regarding involuntary hospitalization, confidentiality, and discrimination. This shows that a law is a starting point for interpretive struggle.

Public participation in medical legislation should include people who experience the system, not only institutional representatives. Protocols, drafts, and reasons should be accessible so that meaningful participation is possible.

5. The National Health Insurance Law as Conceptual Preparation

Key source: National Health Insurance Law, 5754-1994.

The National Health Insurance Law of 1994 established a language of justice, equality, and mutual assistance, thereby creating a social context for the Patients' Rights Law that followed. It regulated compulsory insurance, a benefits basket, and health-fund responsibilities, and was intended to address financial crisis and uneven coverage. Its importance here is not only financial: it moved questions of entitlement into a more explicit public framework, to which the 1996 law could add rights concerning the encounter and the process of care.

In organizational design, the law is not merely a financing mechanism. It defines relations among resident, health fund, and state and permits appeal and legal action. At the same time, updating the benefits basket and budgeting remain arenas of distributive conflict. A medication outside the basket, for example, marks the boundary between individual need and public decision-making. Patients' rights do not automatically compel funding, but they do require a transparent, equal, and reasoned process.

A complementary private market can expand choice but can also create a two-tier system. When availability in the public system erodes, private choice is no longer an addition but a condition for receiving timely care. In Israel, the 1994 and 1996 laws complement one another: the first addresses entitlement and organization more directly, while the second addresses treatment relations and procedure. Separating them narrows the concept of a right.

Every reform should be assessed through two questions: is the service accessible and equal, and is it delivered with dignity, information, and consent? Success in one dimension does not necessarily compensate for failure in the other.

Mechanism of Change: From Private Experience to Legal Rule

A private injury does not become law by itself. Documentation, legal language, a public coalition, examination of data, and a mechanism capable of turning a single story into a rule applicable to other cases are required. This section follows that process of translation and identifies the points at which it can fail.

When private experience becomes a public question: for many years, medical failures were discussed mainly in the language of professionalism and negligence. An injured patient had to show that the physician departed from the standard or caused damage. Gradually it became clear that some injuries are not exhausted by the clinical outcome: concealment of a diagnosis, treatment without consent, disclosure of information, or humiliating treatment. Public criticism transformed such events from personal stories into a discussion of power relations. The very ability to tell the experience outside the institution changed the balance because the system was no longer the only body defining what had happened and what counted as proper. The same act may be experienced differently by someone carrying stigma, dependent on a companion, or afraid of disclosure. These struggles expanded the concept of rights beyond the prohibition of bodily injury. They demanded accessibility, privacy, participation, and nondiscrimination. Their contribution was not only political pressure; they supplied knowledge that the medical record did not produce - how procedures operate in practice and who remains outside services even when formally entitled to them. Case law gradually contributed to recognition that consent is not a courtesy granted by the physician but a condition of the legitimacy of treatment. Claims involving information, confidentiality, and medical battery created a language in which the body is not at the expert's disposal merely because the expert seeks to benefit the patient. Yet a judgment addresses an event that has already occurred and may arrive years later. It can compensate and establish a principle, but it does not necessarily give the care team a tool for handling a disagreement tomorrow morning. Hence the need to move from legal doctrine to a clear organizational framework.

From abstract dignity to an operational right: human dignity provides a guiding principle, but by itself it does not specify what information must be provided, who may inspect a record, or how to act in an emergency. Moving from principle to right requires detail: identifying the harm, defining the duty, establishing exceptions, and creating an enforcement route. Without these steps, dignity remains declaratory language that can be interpreted in contradictory ways.

Case law can accelerate this clarification through a concrete case, but it does not replace legislation, budget, and procedure. A rule born in court should also be tested against situations that never reach litigation and against groups that cannot conduct legal proceedings. Full legitimacy is created when institutions translate the principle into consistent rules and explain their boundaries to the public.

A Coalition That Translates Criticism into a Bill

Public criticism becomes effective when patient organizations, professionals, lawyers, and legislators jointly formulate a common problem. The coalition must decide what belongs in the statute, what remains in procedure, and what requires a budget. Agreement that is too broad can create vague language; excessive detail can freeze a solution that does not fit every situation.

An important stage is early testing: examining a form, procedure, or complaint mechanism in several institutions before general legislation. Such a pilot exposes costs, resistance, and exceptions and allows the law to rest on implementation capacity rather than worthy intention alone.

What makes a law legitimate and workable: legislation requires compromise. Language that is too broad may promise rights the system cannot realize; language that is too narrow may entrench a low standard. The quality of the arrangement is assessed not only by its words but by its mechanisms: who explains, who supervises, what the exception is, how a complaint is received, and what remedy is available. Professional participation matters because professionals know the conditions of work, but those who hold power should not have a veto over the very existence of protection. The claim that rights can weaken trust is not baseless if the law is implemented through forms, threats, and the treatment of every conversation as legal risk. Yet trust without the possibility of review depends on unequal power. A good law does not replace the relationship; it sets a floor that allows the relationship to function. A patient can entrust authority to a physician precisely because the patient knows there are limits, explanations, and a route for correction. Staff can act confidently when exceptions are clear and the institution does not leave them alone facing an impossible demand. To assess the effect of legislation, one must look beyond the number of lawsuits. An increase in complaints may indicate failure, but it may also indicate better accessibility.

A decrease may reflect improvement or fear. Data on information, consent, privacy, response times, and disparities between groups should therefore be combined with interviews and case stories. It is especially important to ask who does not complain: someone who does not speak Hebrew, someone dependent on the same institution, or someone afraid that treatment will be harmed. The law succeeds when these people too can use it without entering a long legal process. The catalysts for legislation teach that durable change grows out of an alliance among law, profession, and public. Without staff, the law may remain impossible to implement; without the public, it may mainly reflect institutional convenience; and without law, protection remains dependent on goodwill. The alliance does not eliminate disagreement but organizes it. It defines what is prohibited, where discretion is required, and who reviews the decision. The literary and social meaning of the transition is a change in the figure of the patient: a rights-bearing person acting within a public institution constrained by resources. The law must protect that person's voice while also explaining limits honestly. When a service is unavailable, a reasoned answer and route of appeal are not substitutes for care, but they prevent scarcity from becoming opacity and arbitrariness.

Communication Between Exposure and System Review

A media report can give voice to a person the system did not hear and place a failure on the public agenda. It also tends to favor an exceptional case, a clear protagonist, and an unambiguous outcome. For a story to become reform rather than only a public storm, it is necessary to ask whether it reveals a pattern: how many similar cases exist, which procedures operated, and what prevented earlier correction.

A responsible institutional response is not limited to protecting reputation and does not immediately adopt the media framing.

It should publish facts that can be disclosed, open an independent review, and report what changed. In this way the media remain a mechanism of exposure, while responsibility for drawing conclusions rests on broader evidence.

Case Law Between the Private Case and the Public Rule

A court decides a concrete dispute, but its reasoning can change the language of an entire system. Recognition of autonomy and dignity broadens the view beyond bodily harm. Yet case law does not plan staffing or queues. When an institution responds only by adding a form, it reduces a human principle to a document. Proper legal translation requires understanding what the rule sought to protect and examining the workflow. Sometimes a change in conversation, information, or responsibility matters more than another page to sign. Reliance on litigation alone creates inequality. Those with time, knowledge, and resources reach court; others give up. Accessible internal and external mechanisms should allow early correction. A judgment can establish a floor and clarify a boundary, but a good complaints system turns that boundary into routine practice. Publishing anonymized decisions and lessons helps teams learn without waiting for the next dispute.

Testing the impact of case law: a judgment can create a principle, but its influence depends on dissemination and implementation. If only lawyers know the doctrine, it will appear in litigation rather than in conversation. The Ministry of Health, professional organizations, and training institutions should translate the principle into scenarios, procedures, and working tools. Recognition of injury to autonomy, for example, should lead to questions about when information was provided and how understanding was checked, not merely another clause on a form. Monitoring changes in practice matters more than counting citations in judgments. Unintended outcomes should also be examined. A legal duty may lead to information overload, overprotection, or avoidance of risky but necessary treatment. That is not a reason to abolish the duty, but to design its implementation carefully. Interviews with patients and staff can show whether change improved dialogue or created ritual. If the form grew longer but understanding did not improve, the problem is not the right but the way it was translated into practice. Law must remain open to learning from implementation.

Groups That Do Not Reach Court

The development of rights through lawsuits can favor people with time, money, and knowledge. People in peripheral regions, immigrants, or dependent patients may never file a claim despite having been harmed. Legislation should therefore also draw on complaint data, ombuds institutions, and community organizations. A short administrative route can surface issues that will never reach court. Publication of anonymized decisions helps staff learn and allows the public to understand the standard. In this way constitutional language does not remain the property of people who have representation. To evaluate equality, one should examine not only how many complaints were received but from which groups and at which stage they dropped out. A person who received a response only after a lawyer intervened points to an inaccessible pathway. Measures can include time, the need for mediation, and whether correction arrived in time. These data connect law with reality and show whether the right protects the weaker person or mainly strengthens those already able to demand.

A Complaint That Arrives Before a Lawsuit

Instead of giving a generic legal answer, the institution appoints a reviewer who collects the record and speaks with both staff and patient. It becomes clear that the conversation took place but in language that was not sufficiently understood. The institution apologizes, assists with continued treatment, and changes its interpreting procedure. The case does not prove that every dispute can be resolved without law, but it shows what an early route can achieve. The response matters even when facts remain disputed. The institution can explain what was found and what cannot be determined without dismissing the experience. Publishing an anonymized lesson allows other institutions to learn. The transition from a language of benevolence to a language of rights also created fear of lost trust. In fact, blind trust is not the goal of a democratic system. Stable trust is created when authority is open to questions, acknowledges limitations, and provides a route for correction. Criticism is not the opposite of professionalism; it is a mechanism that allows professionalism to renew itself. When an institution responds to criticism with data and change, it is not weakened; it shows that it is worthy of the power entrusted to it.

For constitutional language to affect routine practice, schools of medicine, nursing, and management should teach cases and not only statutory sections. Practice in conversation, privacy, and complaints shows how dignity operates under pressure. Managers need tools to translate case law into processes, and lawyers need familiarity with clinical reality. The connection between professions reduces two errors: law that assumes unlimited resources and medicine that treats every demand as legalism. Rights become established when they become a shared language rather than the domain of one specialist. The test case ends not when the Knesset votes, but when the principle reaches the treatment room. If the patient receives information in time, the staff know how to act during disagreement, and a complaint is reviewed before harm becomes irreversible, public criticism has become a living framework. If only a form remains, the law preserves the language of rights but not their meaning. The challenge is to use law to enable better conversation, not replace it.

A patient's complaint that a diagnosis was disclosed in a corridor is initially dismissed as an isolated event. When the complaints officer codes similar complaints by location and time, it becomes clear that they cluster on a shift when the consultation room is being used for storage. The individual story triggered review, but the data identified the mechanism. Instead of simply instructing staff to "be more sensitive," management changes the use of the room and the shift arrangement. This is the difference between a general moral response and a reform whose effect can be tested.

Ombuds Institutions and Complaints as Precursors to Legislation

Before a new law takes shape, accumulated complaints can expose a pattern that case law and the media see only partially. An independent ombuds office can classify complaints, identify recurring failure, and require the institution to respond within a fixed time. Its advantage is relative accessibility and the ability to propose correction without requiring full litigation.

For complaints to become public knowledge, uniform classification and publication of cross-system reports are required. A number alone is insufficient: the type of failure, affected groups, response time, and whether the recommendation was implemented should be reported. An ombuds office that cannot follow correction becomes a mailbox; one with authority to recommend and report to the public can drive change even before the legislature acts.

Such reports also assist in drafting law. They show where a professional rule is insufficient, which exceptions recur, and what the operational cost of the solution is. Legislation can then rest on accumulated experience rather than only on a dramatic case.

Draft, Committee, and Compromise: a bill moves from a moral idea to legal language that institutions must carry out. A committee hears patients, physicians, managers, lawyers, and government ministries. Each group identifies a different risk: harm to autonomy, workload, legal liability, cost, or difficulty in emergencies. Compromise is not necessarily abandonment of principle; sometimes it is how exceptions are defined and a sustainable mechanism is created.

One danger is language so broad that it declares a right without identifying responsibility. Another is rigid detail that does not fit the variety of clinical situations. Good legislation combines a clear principle, authority to issue procedures, judicial review, and a mechanism for updating. It also distinguishes an immediate duty from a goal requiring budget and maturation.

After approval, an implementation period is required: training, adaptation of forms, changes to information systems, and public communication. If this stage is not funded, the law may be perceived as an external threat and function only where a committed manager happens to exist. The quality of legislation is therefore also assessed by its transition plan.

Patient Organizations, AIDS, and the Transformation of Experience into Public Knowledge

Patient organizations changed legislation not only through lawsuits but by creating knowledge. Activists collected testimonies, translated medical information, compared institutions, and showed that a failure that appeared personal recurred among many people. In this way, a public language of accessibility, confidentiality, participation in research, and the right to receive timely explanation emerged.

AIDS activism illustrated both the power and risk of visibility. On one hand, patients and activists demanded rapid access to treatment, participation in research design, and an end to stigma. On the other, disclosure of a diagnosis could damage employment, family relationships, and personal safety. The demand for a right to information therefore went together with a demand for control over information.

An effective patient organization is not merely a pressure group asking for more resources. It can identify a side effect, propose a measure of treatment experience, and test whether a form is understandable. For participation to be legitimate, funding should be disclosed, one group should not be presented as representing all patients, and unorganized voices should also be included.

The legislative lesson is that experience is not an anecdote when it is collected systematically and examined alongside data. A public committee can hear testimony together with professional evidence, ask what pattern it reveals, and translate that pattern into a clear duty. In this way the patient's voice becomes a source of knowledge without replacing scientific evidence.

Professional Codes as Early Reform - and Their Limits

Before detailed legislation, health professions tried to regulate themselves through oaths, codes, and disciplinary rules. A professional code can respond quickly, speak in clinical language, and educate before conflict occurs. It can also set a standard higher than the legal minimum, for example regarding empathy, disclosure of error, or conduct among colleagues.

Self-regulation nevertheless has an inherent conflict. Peers understand the complexity of work, but they may protect the profession's reputation, minimize the patient's experience, or act slowly. When the process is closed and the remedy is not explained, even a sound professional decision struggles to generate trust.

A code becomes meaningful when connected to training, a complaint address, publication of principles, and a fair disciplinary process. It is important to distinguish an error from which learning is possible, behavior that recurs despite training, and intentional misconduct. A uniform response to all situations encourages concealment and does not protect the public more effectively.

Legislation should not replace the professional code but establish a floor, independence, and review. The profession can specify how the duty is implemented, and the public should know who reviews the conduct and what can be done if internal supervision fails. The connection between the two explains how professional change prepared the ground for law but could not substitute for it.

From Private Harm to Binding Change

Channel	**What It Reveals**	**Limitation**	**Condition for Turning the Finding into Reform**
Institutional complaint	Operational failure close to the event	Dependence on the body being reviewed	Documented response and system-wide learning
Media	An experience the system did not see	Tendency toward simplification and exceptional cases	Examination of data alongside the story
Case law	A legal principle arising from a case	Limited access to court	Translation of the judgment into procedure and resources
Public organization	A pattern recurring within a group	Partial representation of the public	Participation of populations that are not organized
Legislation	A binding floor for the entire system	Risk of declaration without implementation	Definition of responsibility, timelines, and oversight

High-quality legal change does not begin with a headline and does not end with publication of a statute. It is built when different channels validate one another: the story signals the harm, the data show its scale, the law formulates a boundary, and the organization receives tools and budget for implementation. Without this chain, a public achievement may remain largely symbolic.

Chapter Six: The Birth of the Patients' Rights Law, 1996 - Legal and Conceptual Analysis

Opening Dilemma

An invasive procedure is scheduled weeks in advance, yet the full explanation is sometimes given only on the morning of the procedure, when the patient is fasting, dressed in hospital clothing, and dependent on the system. Even if a form is signed, freedom of choice is constrained. Genuine implementation requires providing material information as early as possible, allowing questions and a second opinion, and briefly reconfirming consent on the day of the procedure. If the plan has changed, it is necessary to distinguish an unforeseen urgent need from an expansion that could have been discussed in advance. Documentation should reflect the alternatives and the boundaries of consent, not only the name of the procedure. The law does not require every minor risk to be presented with the same intensity.

The law does not give medicine less authority; it requires medicine to justify its authority before the person.

The Patients' Rights Law created in Israel a framework that was relatively comprehensive for its time, combining a right to proper medical treatment, nondiscrimination, informed consent, privacy, information, and the medical record with mechanisms for emergencies and conflict.

Guide to Reading the Legal Chapter

Label	Meaning
Existing law	A rule anchored in statute, case law, or another binding arrangement, as applicable.
Implementation and limits	The gap between the wording of the

Label	Meaning
	right and its operation within an institution, including exceptions, interpretation, and resource conditions.
Proposed direction	The author's recommendation for organizational, regulatory, or legislative change; it should not be read as a description of current law.

This division is intended to help readers who are not lawyers distinguish between what the system is currently required to do and proposals for improvement. In every individual case, the current wording of the law and the circumstances should be examined.

1. Purpose of the Law and the Right to Proper Medical Treatment

Key sources: Patients' Rights Law, 5756-1996, Sections 1 and 5.

Existing law - the purpose clause and the right to proper medical treatment place dignity and privacy alongside professional standards and humane relations, thereby rejecting a separation between clinical quality and human experience. Historically, the law was passed by the Knesset on May 1, 1996, after a prolonged legislative process. It was intended to regulate the rights of people seeking or receiving medical treatment and to protect their dignity and privacy.

Implementation and limits - in practice, proper treatment includes both professional quality and humane relations. This wording matters: a system cannot claim that treatment was good merely because the technical procedure succeeded if the person was humiliated or left without information. A patient who received the correct medication but was spoken to contemptuously and exposed unnecessarily experienced harm that is not cosmetic. Dignity and privacy are part of quality, not additions after the medical work is complete.

At the same time, the term "proper" is open to interpretation and depends on professional standards and resources. That openness allows adaptation over time, but makes direct enforcement and the setting of a clear threshold more difficult. In Israel, within a crowded public system, humane relations are sometimes treated as a personal matter. The law also imposes responsibility on the institution to ensure conditions that make privacy, continuity, and communication possible.

Proposed direction - quality indicators should include explanation, pain management, privacy, respectful treatment, and participation in decisions. An organization that measures only infections, mortality, and length of stay misses part of the legal duty.

2. Nondiscrimination, Emergency Treatment, and Continuity

Existing law - the law seeks to ensure that access to treatment is not denied for improper reasons and that emergency situations do not become occasions for checking entitlement before saving life. The nondiscrimination provisions were drafted within a changing social framework and were later amended and expanded. The right to emergency treatment reflects the ancient principle of rescue and parallels arrangements in other countries.

Implementation and limits - in practice, nondiscrimination is tested not only by an explicit refusal but also by physical accessibility, appointment availability, language, and procedures that create indirect barriers. Continuity requires transfer of information and an appropriate referral when a caregiver stops treatment. Discharging a complex patient without a clear summary and without coordination with community care, for example, may violate the spirit of continuity even if the medical procedure itself was performed correctly. Transitions between institutions are especially vulnerable moments.

Not every distinction is discrimination. Medical triage distinguishes according to urgency and expected benefit. The difficulty is ensuring that the criteria are clinical, transparent, and consistent rather than influenced by stereotypes. Geographic and social disparities in Israel require nondiscrimination to be understood as an active policy. Formal equality at the door is insufficient if waiting time or distance makes the service inaccessible.

Proposed direction - procedures should undergo equality-impact review, waiting times should be published by region and group, accessibility should be ensured, and a rapid mechanism should address allegations of discrimination.

3. Informed Consent: The Core of Autonomy

Key sources: Patients' Rights Law, 5756-1996, Sections 13-15.

Existing law - Sections 13-15 are at the heart of the revolution: treatment requires consent based on information, subject to narrow exceptions balancing the person's wishes with urgency and the need to save life. Historically, the statute specifies information on diagnosis, prognosis, the nature of the procedure, benefit, risks, alternatives, and the risks of no treatment. It requires special forms of consent for certain treatments and recognizes circumstances in which consent cannot be obtained.

Within the institutional framework, an ethics committee may authorize treatment against a patient's wishes under defined conditions, including serious danger, full information, and a reasonable expectation that the patient would consent retrospectively. This is a difficult exception that requires narrow interpretation. A patient who opposes treatment because of fear while the condition deteriorates presents a dilemma between respecting refusal and assessing capacity and understanding. Lack of agreement does not establish incapacity; the person's ability to understand, weigh, and express a choice must be examined.

Implementation and limits - in practice, the signature on a form can become an institutional defense. The law requires information to be provided as early as possible and in a manner that permits voluntary decision-making, not a signature minutes before a procedure when the patient is already dependent and frightened. In Israel, the Daaka judgment strengthened autonomy and recognized compensation for the deprivation of choice itself. Over time, case law sought to define the boundaries of this head of damage so as to prevent double recovery and unlimited expansion.

Proposed direction - the form should be separated from the conversation, tools for checking understanding should be embedded, and preferences should be documented. Complex situations should involve a multidisciplinary team and allow time for a second opinion.

4. The Medical Record, the Right of Access, and Confidentiality

Key sources: Patients' Rights Law, 5756-1996, Sections 17-20.

Existing law - the statute transformed the record from an internal institutional document into a source of information the patient is entitled to inspect, while preserving confidentiality and limited disclosure arrangements. Historically, Section 17 imposes a duty to keep a medical record, Section 18 grants a right to receive information from it, and Sections 19-20 regulate confidentiality and disclosure. The exceptions seek to prevent serious harm or permit essential uses.

Implementation and limits - within the system, a good record supports treatment, safety, continuity, and review. Yet it can be written in judgmental language or contain information about third parties. The right of access therefore also requires professionalism in writing. A patient who discovers an inaccurate label in the record, for example, may suffer its effects for years. The ability to obtain a copy and request correction or the addition of the patient's version is a mechanism of control and identity, not merely a technical matter.

Disclosure of every working note may in rare cases harm a third party or the patient, but broad use of an exception would empty the right of meaning. A decision to withhold information should be reasoned and reviewable. In Israel, online medical records have made access faster, but the scope of sharing has also grown. Genetic information, mental-health data, and application data require updated interpretation and legislation.

Proposed direction - time limits for disclosure, reasonable costs, an accessible interface, and logs of every access to information should be established. Secondary use of data should be secure, proportionate, and transparent to the public.

5. Ethics Committees, Enforcement, and the Gap Between Declaration and Implementation

Key sources: Patients' Rights Law, 5756-1996, Sections 24-25.

Existing law - the law created decision-making mechanisms for sensitive situations, but their strength depends on awareness, availability, independence, and a real ability of patients and staff to approach them. Ethics committees were authorized to consider treatment against a patient's wishes, disclosure of information, and other matters. They were intended to provide solutions close to the time of care rather than waiting for lengthy litigation.

Implementation and limits - institutionally, an internal committee may be too close to management, while an external committee may be too slow. Diverse composition, conflict-of-interest rules, documentation, and accessibility to all parties are required. If a patient or family does not know the committee exists, the right to approach it is theoretical. An employee who fears retaliation will likewise avoid raising a concern even when identifying harm.

The law does not necessarily create a separate cause of action for every violation, and enforcement is dispersed among tort law, discipline, regulation, and public complaints. This dispersion permits flexibility but may weaken deterrence. In Israel, three decades after enactment, implementation is as important as the wording of the sections. Many patients know the phrase "patients' rights" but do not know who is responsible for realizing those rights in real time.

Map of Remedies: From Immediate Decision to Systemic Correction

Not every rights violation requires the same route. A disagreement arising during treatment - for example about information disclosure, refusal of treatment, or family involvement - needs an address capable of acting within hours rather than months. By contrast, a complaint about attitude, delay, or process failure may be handled through public complaints; suspected serious professional misconduct requires disciplinary or regulatory review; and a civil claim deals mainly with compensation and proof of harm. Distinguishing the routes prevents an ethics committee from being asked to decide compensation, or prolonged litigation from substituting for an urgent clinical solution.

An effective mechanism should give the patient a single point of entry even when several bodies operate behind it. The complainant should receive confirmation of receipt, an explanation of who is handling the matter, a timetable, and a reasoned decision. When the decision can still be changed, temporary relief should be considered: postponement of a nonurgent procedure, a second opinion, immediate access to documents, or urgent ethics-committee review. This preserves the possibility of correction before the right becomes merely a retrospective debate.

The final stage is returning the lesson to the system. A complaint that ends with a private apology is insufficient if the same failure recurs in other departments. Complaints should be coded by subject, patterns identified, anonymized findings published, and responsibility for change assigned. At the same time, staff and patients who report problems in good faith require protection so that the mechanism does not encourage silence. In this way, enforcement is not viewed only as legal threat but as a route for resolution, learning, and prevention.

Proposed direction - activity reports of ethics committees should be published, an independent patients' rights ombuds institution should be created or existing mechanisms strengthened, whistleblowers should be protected, and periodic training should be required for all employees.

Operationalizing the Law: From Right to Practical Remedy

A right is useful only when it is clear who is authorized to act, within what time, and what happens if the request is unanswered. The practical focus is matching the response route to the type of harm - postponing an action, completing information, obtaining record access, approaching an ethics committee, or making an organizational correction.

Planning Consent Before the Last Moment

When the conversation takes place minutes before a procedure, freedom of choice is reduced even if all information is technically provided. Proper planning identifies complex decisions in advance, sends adapted material, allows questions, and separates the time of explanation from the time of signature. When there is no medical urgency, scheduling pressure is not a reason to shorten the process.

The record should document alternatives and questions that remain open and identify who is responsible for returning to the patient. Consent thereby becomes a continuing process of clarification rather than a ritual beside the operating room.

Disclosure to a Third Party: Graduated Authorization and Use Control

A patient may decide who receives information on the patient's behalf, but authorization should not be broader than necessary. A distinction can be drawn between a companion who may receive verbal updates, a power of attorney authorized to receive documents, and a professional who receives information for a defined action. This distinction is especially important in prolonged illness, when a family member who was involved during hospitalization is not necessarily the person the patient wishes to involve in every future visit.

Authorization should be amendable and revocable and recorded in a form the team can understand in real time. When the patient cannot express a view, only information necessary for treatment or protection of an essential interest should be disclosed, not the entire file. A sound information system shows who received authorization, for what purpose, and until when, and documents exceptional disclosures. Confidentiality therefore does not obstruct continuity, but neither is it breached simply because someone is a relative.

The Ethics Committee as an Operational Service

An ethics committee is useful only if it can be reached while the decision is still open. An institution should define on-call availability, a short referral route, and a composition capable of hearing the patient, family, and team. The committee is not a small court; its role is to map the values, clarify the facts, and propose a reasoned course of action.

After the decision, the underlying principle should be documented and disseminated anonymously. In this way, a single case improves the ability of departments to handle a similar dispute without turning every event into a rigid precedent.

Complaint and Remedy Routes That Do Not Depend on Litigation

A sick person is not always able to conduct legal proceedings. Litigation may arrive years after the event, when the immediate goal was to receive an explanation, correct a record, or prevent discontinuation of care. A sequence of accessible addresses is therefore needed: a departmental contact, an institutional officer, and an external ombuds body. Multiple uncoordinated addresses confuse patients and shift the burden onto them. A single entry point that routes the matter can preserve internal expertise without requiring the person to know in advance who is responsible. To use such a system well, it is necessary to distinguish an isolated incident from a pattern, dissatisfaction from a rights violation, and a local problem from a failure at the interface between organizations. A good response is not limited to rejection or a general apology. It explains what was examined, what was corrected, and what the complainant can do if dissatisfied. Staff are also entitled to a fair process and an opportunity to present their position. A system that punishes every error will encourage concealment, but a system that never assigns responsibility will deepen mistrust. Measurement of implementation should focus on meaningful decisions: when information was provided, whether an alternative was presented, whether an interpreter was used, how long it took to obtain a record, and the response time of an ethics committee or urgent complaint. Data should be stratified by institution type, time, and language.

A right available only during business hours is not sufficient in an emergency department. A complex institution serving a vulnerable population may report more complaints, and that may reflect accessibility rather than poor quality. Joint training for physicians, nurses, managers, and reception staff is essential because rights begin before the clinical conversation. Inaccessible scheduling, an incomprehensible form, or a clerk who does not know where to refer a person can empty the law of meaning. Practice should be based on real cases: a change in a procedure plan, a family request to conceal information, refusal, access to the record, or a complaint during a busy shift. This allows employees to see the law as a decision-making tool rather than an external threat. A living law is measured by whether it changes the division of labor. If consent requires time, the system must allocate that time earlier; if there is a right to an opinion, record transfer must be enabled; if an ethics committee exists, it must be accessible. The entire duty cannot be placed on the physician at the last moment while the organization remains outside the picture. Responsibility grows with control over resources and processes. The patient is expected to provide information and respect staff, but the institution sets the conditions in which this is possible.

Privacy During a Busy Shift

Workload does not abolish privacy, but it requires realistic solutions. A curtain, lowering one's voice, checking identity before disclosing information, and avoiding sensitive conversations in a corridor are simple steps. When no room is available, the limitation should be explained and the best possible location chosen. Telephone conversations require identity verification and consent before information is given to a relative. Privacy breaches sometimes arise from habit rather than intent. A brief observation and team discussion can identify recurring points: an exposed screen, a printed list, or calling a full name aloud. General annual training is not enough. Environmental changes - screen filters, headphones, and a designated place for conversation - can help more than exhortation. The organization is responsible for creating conditions, and the worker is responsible for using them.

Confidentiality Versus Continuity and the Welfare of Others

When information is disclosed to save another person, for public health, or under an order, the scope should be minimized and the justification documented. The team should know when legal authorization is required and when action can be taken under a professional duty. Uncertainty sometimes leads to excessive sharing or to concealment that creates danger. Accessible privacy consultation can prevent both extremes. Where possible, the patient should be informed of the disclosure and its limits. A corridor conversation, an open screen, or calling out a name are also privacy events. The law does not deal only with large databases. Spatial design, screen locking, and conversation rules are part of implementation. A crowded ward may not always have a private room, but staff can move away, lower their voices, and determine what information is necessary. Small intrusions repeated every day can erode trust no less than an exceptional event. Privacy review should include observation of routine practice and not only investigation after a leak.

When the Right Arrives at the Wrong Time: much healthcare takes place at night, on weekends, and on holidays. A right to an ethics committee, an interpreter, or urgent access to a record is insufficient if the service is available only during office hours. It is not necessary to maintain every mechanism in full at all hours, but on-call coverage, remote consultation, and an escalation route are required. The institution should examine whether exceptional decisions are made more frequently during hours when support is absent. A permanent day-night gap is a quality and rights problem, not merely an operational issue. A junior employee on a night shift may be left facing an angry family and a dispute the employee lacks authority to resolve. The patient also needs to know when a final answer will be given and what will happen in the meantime. Temporariness must be defined; "we will check tomorrow" is insufficient when treatment is changing now. The division of responsibility among the on-duty clinician, on-call senior staff, and management is part of the living law.

Organizational Proofreading of Forms and Procedures: before adding a new form, existing documents should be mapped.

Duplication creates burden and hides the important question. Information can be consolidated, language shortened, and explanatory material separated from documentation of consent. A good form supports a conversation and does not attempt to contain every scenario. Testing with patients and staff can identify unclear terms and fields no one uses. Linguistic editing of the document thereby becomes editing of the process itself. The law should appear in training through cases, not only lectures. Teams can analyze a failed conversation, identify where explanation was needed, and ask what could have been done differently. Multidisciplinary learning prevents each field from seeing only its own part. When law is integrated into clinical work, it ceases to be a threat and helps decision-making. This is a condition for the framework to remain alive after the initial excitement of enactment has passed.

Urgent Transfer of Information Between Institutions

When care moves to another institution, information required for decision-making should arrive before or with the patient. There is no need to open the entire record: a clinical summary, relevant tests, medication list, allergies, and unresolved decisions should be transferred. The sending institution verifies the recipient's identity and the delivery channel; the receiving institution confirms that the material was received and is readable. If an essential document is missing, a professional contact should be established to complete it rather than returning the patient to an ordinary bureaucratic route. Urgent transfer also requires an explanation to the person: what was sent, to whom, and why. After the event, it can be examined whether the urgent request reflected a genuine exception or a recurring failure in referral. This prevents an emergency mechanism from becoming a privacy bypass while also ensuring that confidentiality does not obstruct timely safe care.

A patient is referred on a Friday evening for urgent surgery at another center, but the imaging study is stored in a system that is not connected. An authorized on-call employee generates a secure time-limited link, transfers it directly to the receiving team, and documents the action. On the next business day, the institution examines why the referral did not include the material from the outset. Distinguishing immediate solution from root correction prevents two errors: delaying treatment in the name of a rigid procedure, and turning the exception into uncontrolled information disclosure.

Graduated Administrative Enforcement: not every violation requires litigation, but the absence of a consistent response erodes the law. Administrative enforcement can begin with a correction requirement, progress to an action plan and repeat audit, and reach sanctions when failure is serious or persistent. Such a ladder distinguishes an isolated error from an organizational pattern.

The process should be transparent: the institution knows what is required, within what time, and what will happen if the requirement is not met. In matters of public interest, anonymized findings and system-wide recommendations may be published. Publication is not intended to shame but to demonstrate that the law is being implemented and to prevent every organization from learning only from its own mistakes.

Good enforcement also examines resources. If a violation stems from an information system that does not permit access or from the absence of interpreting, structural correction is required rather than employee training alone. Responsibility remains with the institution that organizes the service.

Minors and Adults Who Need Support

Rights do not disappear when a person does not have full decision-making capacity. For a minor, parental consent should be combined with age-appropriate explanation and involvement of the child according to age and understanding. The more significant the decision and the more mature the minor, the greater the weight that should be given to the minor's views, with privacy preserved in sensitive matters.

For a person with cognitive difficulty, the specific decision should be assessed rather than relying on diagnosis alone. Simple support - time, plain language, an image, a familiar person, or breaking the decision into stages - may make decision-making possible. Only when support is insufficient does a representative step in, and even then that representative should act in accordance with prior wishes and values, not only personal preferences.

The system should document which adjustments were made and what worked. Such documentation protects against automatic removal of voice and allows the next team to use a communication method already found effective.

A Second Opinion as a Usable Right: a second opinion is not useful if the patient does not know whom to contact, cannot obtain the record, or must wait until the treatment option is no longer available. An institution should explain when a second opinion is relevant, how material is transferred, and what costs are involved. In urgent situations, rapid professional consultation between teams can be arranged rather than placing all organizational burden on the patient.

Negative treatment after requesting a second opinion must also be prevented. Such a request is not a vote of no confidence but a legitimate tool in complex decision-making. When two opinions conflict, the team should explain the basis of disagreement rather than leaving the person to choose between authorities without guidance.

Correcting the Record Without Erasing History

The right of access does not solve the situation in which a patient discovers an incorrect fact, offensive description, or interpretation that continues to affect care. Correction need not erase the original document; deletion may harm the reliability of the record and the ability to understand what information the team had when it made a decision. The proper method is to add a dated correction, identify who made it, and preserve an audit trail.

A distinction should be made between verifiable facts and professional disagreement. An incorrect address, a medication that was not taken, or a surgery that never occurred requires prompt correction. A diagnosis or clinical impression may be disputed; in that situation the patient should be able to add a position, document, or opinion, and the next team should be able to see that the matter is contested. Leaving a label without context can turn an old hypothesis into a permanent identity.

The request mechanism should be simple, with a response time and a route of appeal. A request should not automatically return to the same person who wrote the record when a conflict of interest is possible. In digital systems, it is also necessary to ensure that the correction reaches places where the inaccurate information has already been copied - a referral, discharge summary, or problem list. A local correction that does not reach the next system does not restore the right in practice.

A useful measure is not only the number of corrections but processing time, the proportion of requests partially accepted, and whether corrected information continues to appear in new documents. The record thereby remains reliable professional documentation while not imprisoning the person inside an error no one is willing to review.

Companion and Decision Supporter in the Medical Encounter

The presence of a supportive person can turn a formal right into a practical ability. A patient may remember only part of the explanation, find it difficult to ask questions, or be afraid to disagree. A companion chosen by the patient can take notes, remind the team of preferences, and help after the visit. The role is not to replace the person's voice but to expand the person's ability to participate.

The right to accompaniment is not absolute at every moment. An intimate examination, concern about harm, another person's confidentiality, or actual interference with treatment may justify restriction. The decision should, however, be specific and reasoned rather than a blanket policy excluding families. Before asking a companion to leave, the patient should be asked privately whether the presence is desired and whether the patient feels free to speak.

When the companion takes over the conversation, the team should return the center of gravity to the patient. Staff can address the patient directly, offer part of the conversation in private, and clarify what information may be disclosed. In cases of communication difficulty, a professional interpreter is not automatically replaced by a family member; the companion can support the person but should not carry sole responsibility for accuracy and explanation.

A proper institution sets simple rules in advance: how the patient identifies who may receive information, when presence may be restricted, who has authority to decide a dispute, and how the person's wishes are documented. Accompaniment then ceases to be a favor dependent on an individual staff member and does not become a route around confidentiality.

Operational and Remedy Map by Type of Right

The law becomes alive when each right has a response time, a responsible address, and an appropriate type of remedy. Not every disagreement requires court, but not every injury is resolved by a local apology. A mature system distinguishes among stopping harm, restoring a right, compensation, disciplinary review, and process correction - and connects them without forcing the patient to navigate the entire structure.

Right	**Real-Time Failure**	**Immediate Response**	**Follow-Up Route**
Informed consent	Information provided too close to the procedure	Safe postponement and completion of the conversation	Process review and staff training

Right	**Real-Time Failure**	**Immediate Response**	**Follow-Up Route**
Access to the record	Partial or unreadable material	Disclosure in a usable format with explanation	Complaints officer or appropriate legal process
Confidentiality	Unnecessary disclosure	Stop access and document the event	Authorization review and notice to the affected person
Emergency treatment	Disagreement about capacity or refusal	Senior consultation and proportionate solution	Ethics committee and documentation of reasons
Proper and equal treatment	Service disparity or discrimination	Remove the barrier and ensure continuity	Administrative, regulatory, or judicial review

Part Three: Israel After the Law - Service, Resources, and the Boomerang Effect of Violence

The law changed the language and expectations, but it did not create hospital beds, nursing positions, appointments, or time for conversation. Part Three moves from the normative framework to the emergency department, clinic, and hospital ward. It examines the gap between written rights and the conditions that make their realization possible, as well as the growing awareness of violence against healthcare staff. The possible relationship between patient empowerment and the erosion of authority will be examined cautiously, distinguishing among correlation, causal mechanisms, and alternative explanations.

Chapter Seven: Clinical Reality in the Modern Era - Quality, Accessibility, and the Gap Between Law and Resources

Opening Dilemma

An older patient is discharged after an exacerbation of heart failure. The discharge summary lists new medications, a blood test within three days, and an appointment with a cardiologist. At home, it becomes clear that the prescription does not match the medications already in his possession, the laboratory will not accept the referral, and the first available appointment is two months away. His daughter calls several service centers and receives different answers. A week later, he returns to the emergency department. Each action, viewed separately, appeared reasonable; the failure arose between them. Proper planning would have included medication reconciliation at the bedside, scheduling the test before discharge, transmitting the summary to community care, and a brief follow-up call. The scenario shows why handing over a document is not equivalent to transferring responsibility. Discharge instructions should focus on changes: what was stopped, what was added, which symptoms require seeking care, and who will provide an answer.

A respectful conversation cannot take place within a timetable that does not recognize human time.

A right established by law may erode when a system does not provide time, continuity, accessibility, and sufficient staffing; the failure is organizational, not merely a moral failing of the individual caregiver.

1. Rights Under Pressure: Time as an Ethical Resource

Time is a hidden precondition for almost every right: to explain, listen, check understanding, protect privacy, and coordinate continued care. A shortage of time turns formal rights into box-checking exercises. Historically, healthcare systems around the world have had to contend with aging populations, chronic disease, and expensive technologies. In Israel, rapid population growth, disparities between the center and the periphery, and prolonged periods of emergency have added further pressure.

For institutions, productivity indicators encourage shorter visits and earlier discharge. When an organization rewards the number of patients seen rather than the quality of understanding, the caregiver must choose between meeting a target and conducting a complete conversation. An emergency physician, for example, may rapidly provide all legally required information yet fail to notice that the patient did not understand a key term. The signature exists, but the decision is not genuinely informed.

The issue is more complex, however: simply increasing the time allocated to every encounter is not the only solution, and it may reduce accessibility. Tasks should be distributed among team members, advance information should be used, and cases requiring extended time should be identified. In Israel, crowding in emergency departments and internal-medicine wards has become a symbol of the gap between a highly professional system and limited infrastructure. The right to dignity is also harmed when a patient is treated in a corridor without privacy.

Time for explanation should be treated as a funded therapeutic activity. Coordinating nurses, clinical pharmacists, and information tools should be used, and understanding and satisfaction should be measured alongside throughput.

2. Geographic, Financial, and Digital Accessibility

Accessibility is not merely an open door; it is the ability to reach, afford, understand, and use a service at a time appropriate to the medical condition. Historically, the expansion of community services and the shift to digital care improved availability for many people. At the same time, some services were closed or centralized, creating dependence on technology and transportation.

In practice, a long wait in the center of the country, hours of travel from the periphery, a copayment, or an inaccessible digital scheduling system can create indirect discrimination. Entitlement exists, but use is impossible. An older person who does not use a smartphone may miss an appointment or important information. A digital solution that reduces burden for the general public may deepen the exclusion of a vulnerable group.

In the clinical arena, not every advanced service can be maintained in every locality. Concentrating expertise may improve quality. The obligation is to provide transportation, telemedicine, travel reimbursement, and community continuity that counterbalance centralization. In Israel, geographic distances are relatively short compared with large countries, but disparities in infrastructure, transportation, and workforce create real differences among regions. Cultural and linguistic accessibility adds another layer.

Every decision to centralize a service should include an impact assessment, a local alternative, published waiting times, and support for people who are not digitally connected. Accessibility is a matter of planning, not a gesture.

3. Continuity of Care and Transitions Between Organizations

Patients are sometimes harmed not within a particular unit but in the space between hospital and community, specialist and family physician, or healthcare and social services. Medical specialization has produced deep expertise, but also fragmentation. Chronic illness and polypharmacy require long-term coordination that does not fit a model built around a single episode of care.

Within the system, separate information systems, unclear responsibility, and distinct financing incentives impede the transfer of information. Patients sometimes become couriers carrying documents between large organizations. Discharge after hospitalization without a follow-up appointment or medication reconciliation, for example, may lead to readmission. Every unit may claim that it performed its task, while the system as a whole has failed.

Information sharing improves continuity but also raises privacy risks. Access should therefore be granted according to need, documented, and accompanied by a clear explanation to the patient of who is responsible at each stage. Israel's health funds provide a relative advantage in community continuity, but transitions from hospitals under different ownership structures and coordination with social services remain complex.

A timely discharge summary, a handoff conversation, case management for complex patients, and an organizational follow-up target are ways to turn continuity from a general right into identifiable responsibility.

Transition from Hospitalization to Rehabilitation: A Functional Window of Opportunity

After a mild stroke, a patient is found suitable for intensive rehabilitation, but the admission request is sent only on the day of discharge. By the time a response arrives, the rehabilitation bed has been taken and the patient returns to a home that is not adapted to her needs. Here, the failure is not in providing a medication or document, but in losing a window of time in which early practice may affect function, independence, and the ability to return to life in the community.

Rehabilitation planning should begin during hospitalization: functional assessment, review of home conditions, selection of an appropriate setting, and transfer of professional information to the receiving provider. When no place is immediately available, an interim plan is required, including community treatment, equipment, family instruction, and a fixed date for reassessment. It is not enough to write 'rehabilitation recommended' when it is clear that the patient cannot arrange the service alone.

In such a transition, responsibility is measured by functional outcome, not merely by completion of a referral. The system should examine how long it took for rehabilitation to begin, whether an alternative was provided during the waiting period, and whether people from peripheral regions or without family support wait longer. This indicator reveals whether a sound clinical decision became an actual service and prevents a situation in which every organization displays a proper document while the person's functional ability deteriorates.

4. Quality of Service, Errors, and Transparency

Key sources: Institute of Medicine, 2000; WHO, 2021.

Medical quality does not mean the complete absence of errors, but the ability to reduce them, identify them, disclose information, and learn from them without concealment and without turning every failure into a hunt for someone to blame. Historically, the patient-safety movement demonstrated that adverse events often arise from design, communication, and environment rather than from individual negligence alone. Aviation and other industries provided models of reporting and learning.

At the institutional level, a punitive culture encourages concealment, but a culture without accountability undermines trust. A just culture is needed, one that distinguishes among human error, risky behavior, and deliberate violations. Administration of the wrong medication because of similar packaging, workload, and the absence of a double-check requires treatment of the patient, disclosure, support for the team, and correction of the system. Dismissing an employee alone does not prevent the next event.

Openness may increase fear of litigation, but concealment increases anger and harm. Models of disclosure, apology, and fair compensation may reduce escalation and rebuild trust. In Israel, the patient's rights to information and to the medical record provide a foundation for transparency, but disclosure to families is not always consistent. A gap remains between an internal investigation and sharing information with the person who was harmed.

A procedure for disclosure of adverse events should be established, managers should be trained to conduct these conversations, safety reporting should be protected, and aggregate data should be published. Institutional accountability is a condition for rights.

5. Person-Centered Medicine Without Turning the Patient into a Consumer Alone

Respectful service should recognize needs and preferences, but the image of the patient as a customer can distort a system based on professionalism, solidarity, and resource allocation. Historically, the language of service entered healthcare together with satisfaction measures, competition, and choice of provider. It contributed to accessibility and respectful treatment, but it also imported the expectation that the customer is always right.

In practice, a hospital is not a hotel and a physician is not selling a product. A professional decision may include refusing antibiotics, a test, or hospitalization that is not clinically necessary. Good service does not mean agreeing to every request. A patient demanding imaging without an indication, for example, may feel that a right has been denied. A respectful explanation of radiation harm, incidental findings, and alternatives is a realization of rights even when the request is refused.

Opposition to consumerism, however, is not an excuse to return to paternalism. The patient is entitled to influence decisions, ask questions, and challenge them. The distinction is between partnership and a transaction in which payment or loudness determines priority. In Israel, the combination of public medicine, supplementary insurance, and private insurance creates conflicting identities: citizen, insured person, customer, and patient at the same time. The resulting confusion affects expectations and trust.

The language should therefore be one of partnership and health citizenship: clear rights, mutual responsibility, an explanation of limits, and transparent allocation decisions. In this way, service can be improved without commercializing the relationship.

The Patient Journey: Responsibility in Transitions Between Organizations

Most failures of continuity occur not within a single treatment episode but at a transition: a referral that was not recognized, a medication that was not reconciled, equipment that did not arrive, or a message that was not transmitted to community care. This section constructs a pathway of responsibility across organizations and defines how to verify that information and care have actually reached their destination.

The right exists between institutions as well. Healthcare systems are built around organizations: a hospital is responsible for hospitalization, a health fund for community care, a supplier for equipment, and a public authority for social services. The person, by contrast, experiences one illness. When responsibility changes hands, information may disappear and the task may shift to the patient. A discharge letter can be accurate yet fail to lead to an appointment; a prescription can be correct yet never be filled; a referral can be sent without anyone checking whether it was received. The patient need not perform every task, but should know who is responsible for medications, tests, equipment, and follow-up. In a complex hospitalization, that person may be a coordinating nurse; in the community, a family physician or case manager. Assigning ownership does not eliminate the responsibility of others. It prevents every unit from assuming that the next unit will take care of the problem.

The patient should receive a name and a means of contact, not merely a general instruction to contact the health fund. Even when a service is provided by an external supplier, the public body is not relieved of the duty to verify that the referral was carried out. Legally, institutional fragmentation should not create a vacuum. The right to information includes an explanation of who is responsible after discharge and what the warning signs are. Proper care includes reasonable planning of follow-up when the risk is known. Not every delay constitutes a violation of rights, but persistent ambiguity and the inability to obtain an answer can turn scarcity into arbitrariness. The most useful remedy during a transition is often an immediate correction - a prescription, appointment, or piece of equipment - rather than compensation after the fact. A contact mechanism must therefore be able to act in time and route the request among organizations without returning the person to the starting point.

A Referral Rejected Because of an Unclear Criterion

A patient is referred to a pain clinic, but the request is returned with the general explanation 'missing information.' The referring physician does not know which document is required, and the patient discovers the rejection only weeks later. A fair pathway requires clear notice, specification of what is missing, an opportunity to correct the deficiency without opening a new referral, and a date on which the request will be reassessed. When there is a dispute over eligibility for the service, a brief clinical appeal is needed rather than a struggle between service centers. This preserves professional triage without turning an internal criterion into a barrier that no one can understand or correct.

Digital Systems That Connect - and Digital Systems That Exclude: Digital systems make it possible to transmit summaries, results, and appointments quickly. They also create an assumption that the person is connected, can read the message, and understands which document matters. An essential service should retain a human alternative that is not inferior and does not involve unreasonable waiting. An automated message is not confirmation that the information was understood. In a high-risk transition, active verification is required - a conversation, acknowledgment of receipt, or confirmation that the task was completed. Continuity is not a license to transfer the entire medical record to every provider. Only necessary information should be shared, permissions should be defined, and the patient should be told who is involved. When several systems do not communicate with one another, repeated printing and unnecessary exposure should not be justified in the name of efficiency. A good technological solution reduces duplication and allows the professional to see the current plan, but it also records who accessed information and allows errors to be corrected.

Error, Disclosure, and Learning Along the Pathway

When an error in a transition is discovered - an incorrect dose, an appointment that was not scheduled, or information that did not arrive - transparency is part of care. Responsible disclosure includes explaining what is known, immediately addressing any harm, apologizing when appropriate, and providing an update on the steps taken. Ambiguity may protect the institution in the short term, but it deepens the injury. A learning culture should distinguish personal negligence from process failure. An employee who reports a discrepancy in time is not the source of the problem; that employee is a protective mechanism. Learning, however, does not excuse responsibility when disregard or concealment is repeated. A reporting system should link events by care pathway and not merely by department. If several patients return to the emergency department because they did not receive equipment in the community, each case may appear isolated within the hospital and the health fund. Joint analysis reveals the pattern. The system should also examine people who do not return and do not complain - those who abandon treatment, pay privately, or rely on family. The absence of a complaint is not proof that the transition succeeded. Sometimes it means that the person did not know whom to contact.

Measures That Begin with the Outcome Experienced by the Person: Core measures include completion of tests and appointments on time, medication reconciliation, receipt of equipment, preventable readmissions, and understanding of instructions. Results should be stratified by age, language, location, and social circumstances, because an average can conceal a group that repeatedly falls through the cracks. Data should be accompanied by case narratives and conversations with staff to determine whether failures arise from information systems, workforce shortages, or instructions that cannot be implemented. A single target can produce gaming of the numbers. Pressure to shorten hospitalization may appear successful while simultaneously increasing unsafe discharges. Length of stay should therefore be linked with measures of continuity, safety, and experience. Data need to return to the team quickly. An annual report alone does not help a nurse who notices today that prescriptions are not arriving. An internal dashboard can display open tasks and who is responsible, while public reporting presents trends and disparities among groups. In Israel, where responsibility is divided among hospitals, health funds, institutes, and suppliers, it is possible to begin with high-risk situations: older people with polypharmacy, oncology patients, rehabilitation, and respiratory equipment. Each pathway should have a coordinating professional, a timeframe for follow-up review, and a single point of contact. There is no need to establish a large new body for every patient; existing teams can be used and given permission to view tasks and resolve barriers. The pilot should include central and peripheral regions, Hebrew and additional languages, to ensure that the solution does not depend on a highly capable family or a resource-rich institution.

Medication Reconciliation as Shared Ownership of the Medication List

A medication list is not reliable merely because it appears on a computer screen. During the transition from hospitalization to community care, what was prescribed must be compared with what the patient actually takes, what was discontinued, and what is taken without a prescription. Responsibility should be shared but not ambiguous: one professional consolidates the list, the approving physician resolves discrepancies, and the receiving institution confirms that it received and understood the information.

The patient receives a short document explaining what changed and why, with a way to make contact if a discrepancy arises. The completion measure is not the production of the letter itself, but verification that the list was updated by the next responsible provider and that no duplication or dangerous discontinuation occurred.

A Digital Gateway That Is Not the Only Door

Portals and applications provide access to results, scheduling, and messages. They can also become the only way to reach a service. A person without a smartphone, password, or digital literacy is left behind. A person should not be penalized for failing to open a message sent through a channel that person did not choose. During registration, the service should explain what will be sent and how communication preferences can be updated. Immediate automatic publication can strengthen autonomy, but it can also leave a person alone with difficult information. An explanation, a contact number, and a time when a professional will call back can be added. The solution is to distinguish among types of information and allow choice. The system should document who is responsible for follow-up and should not assume that viewing a result is equivalent to understanding it.

Home Care and the Boundary Between Family and System

Moving care into the home can improve quality of life and prevent hospitalization, but it also transfers work to the family. Before discharge, the system should determine who is available, what that person's abilities are, and what burden is involved. Instruction should include practice, not merely a handout. Equipment should arrive before the patient, and a point of contact should be available in the evening as well. When the family cannot provide the necessary support, this should not be presented as a lack of commitment; a professional or community solution is required. The family caregiver also needs protection. The system should ask whether that person agrees to assume the role, allow respite, and identify burnout. The patient's privacy continues at home; information should be shared with a family member according to authorization. When several relatives are involved, it is useful to designate a contact person without excluding the others. Successful home care connects professionalism with support and does not treat family closeness as a free resource.

Transitions in Which Continuity Requires More Than a Discharge Letter

A child moving to adult services, a person discharged from psychiatric hospitalization, and a patient beginning rehabilitation all require a tailored pathway. In each case, the professionals, language of service, and degree of family responsibility change. A transition meeting, a designated professional, and a period during which both services remain available should therefore be established.

Continuity also includes equipment, social rights, and the ability to reach treatment. Providing a recommendation without coordinating a device, transportation, or financing leaves responsibility with the person at the most vulnerable moment. The test is whether the next service actually began, not whether the referral was sent.

Waiting and the Right to an Update

The patient journey also includes waiting within community care. A referral that has been sent but receives no response turns the person into the manager of follow-up. A system can send confirmation of receipt, an estimated timeframe, and instructions on what to do if the condition worsens. When an appointment is postponed, the patient should be informed rather than expected to discover the change upon arrival. When an important test is not performed, there should be follow-up on nonattendance. This does not mean pursuing every person, but identifying high-risk situations and determining whether the barrier is language, transportation, or an informed decision. If the person refuses, the refusal should be documented and the door left open. If the person did not know about the appointment, the failure belongs to the system. This distinction prevents patients from being labeled 'noncompliant' when the pathway itself is inaccessible.

Shared Responsibility That Is Not Ambiguous: An agreement between a hospital and a health fund can define the minimum information required, the timeframe for transfer, and a mechanism for resolving discrepancies. There is no need to wait for new legislation to create a standard. Teams on both sides can review recurring cases and repair the interface. When one organization changes a procedure, it should update the other. Continuity thus becomes an organizational agreement rather than the improvisation of a diligent employee. When failure occurs, the patient needs a single point of contact even if responsibility is divided. The body that receives the inquiry should continue to provide updates until the problem has been routed, rather than say, 'That is not our responsibility.' Behind the scenes, the organizations can determine who bears final responsibility. This principle reduces the burden of navigation and also helps staff by defining how a case should be handed off without being lost.

An Abnormal Result That Was Never Closed

A pathology result arrives after the patient has already returned to community care and indicates the need for further investigation. The result appears in the record, but no one is designated to make contact or verify that an appointment was scheduled. Closing the loop requires assigning an owner to every significant result, confirming that the patient received and understood the information, and documenting the action that was decided upon. If contact cannot be made, attempts should be escalated according to the level of risk rather than automatically marking the person as 'no response.' If the person chooses not to continue, an informed choice should be documented and a route back should remain available. In this way, follow-up respects autonomy without turning publication of a result in a digital system into a substitute for clinical responsibility.

In a multi-organizational system, rules are also needed for results that arrive after responsibility has been transferred. The laboratory knows who ordered the test, but the ordering professional may no longer be the active caregiver. A safe mechanism sends the alert both to the ordering professional and to the current clinical address and escalates when receipt is not acknowledged. The important measure is the time from an abnormal result to documented action, together with an examination of who is lost to follow-up because of a change of address, transfer between health funds, or lack of digital access.

Medical Equipment at Home and Responsibility for Instruction: Discharge with an oxygen device, pump, or feeding equipment does not end with handing over a box. The system must verify that the equipment arrived, the home is suitable, the caregiver knows how to use it, and there is a point of contact for malfunctions. Instruction under pressure on the day of discharge is not enough; practice, accessible materials, and confirmation of understanding are required.

Ownership of responsibility should remain clear even when the supplier is external. The patient should not have to mediate among the company, health fund, and hospital department. A malfunction at night requires an emergency route, and a change of model requires renewed instruction. A quality measure can examine malfunctions, repeat contacts, and hospitalizations resulting from incorrect use.

In this way, home equipment becomes part of continuity of care rather than a transfer of risk from the institution to the family.

Telemedicine and Digital Continuity

A video consultation can save travel and allow frequent follow-up, but it is not suitable for every examination or every person. An in-person alternative should be offered, privacy in the home should be considered, and the patient's ability to use the system should be verified. A dropped connection or an inadequate image is not the patient's failure.

Digital continuity requires that the summary enter the shared record, recommendations be transmitted to the treating professional, and the next examination be scheduled. Without such integration, telemedicine creates another channel that does not communicate with the rest of the system. Benefit should be measured not by the number of calls, but by the ability to complete care safely.

Sensory and Cognitive Accessibility That Does Not Depend on a Companion

Medical accessibility is tested even when the person reaches the clinic on time. A patient with hearing loss, blindness, difficulty reading, or cognitive disability may receive the same formal service yet leave without understanding what was decided. Routine reliance on a family member makes the right to information dependent on another person's availability and may also compromise privacy.

An organization should maintain a range of accommodations: assistive listening systems, documents accessible to screen readers, large print, plain-language explanations, symbols, additional time, and the option to record a summary with consent. The accommodation is chosen with the patient, not according to a general label. Two people with the same diagnosis may need different forms of communication, and a person may prefer human assistance to a digital tool.

When cognitive difficulty exists, the decision should be broken into stages and understanding of the specific action should be assessed. Support is not equivalent to replacing the person's will. A companion can help remember information and formulate questions, but the team should also address the patient directly, identify agreement or objection, and document what support enabled participation. This prevents a rapid jump from communication difficulty to a conclusion that the person lacks capacity.

Assessing accessibility requires more than an inventory of equipment. It is possible to measure how many appointments were postponed because a communication accommodation was unavailable, whether visit summaries were provided in an appropriate format, and whether patients could repeat the treatment plan. Such data reveal disparities that are invisible in a waiting-time measure alone.

Return to Life Roles After Initial Rehabilitation

Treatment success is not measured only by the ability to get out of bed, walk down a corridor, or perform a basic task. After the initial rehabilitation phase ends, another test emerges: can the person return to the roles that give life meaning - work, study, parenting, social relationships, and participation in the community? Two people with similar motor outcomes may face entirely different realities because of occupation, transportation, family support, or social attitudes.

The return plan should be developed separately from the rehabilitation admission plan. It includes vocational or educational assessment, physical and technological accommodations, a gradual return, and coordination with the workplace or educational institution - and only with the patient's consent. A person should not be required to disclose medical information that is unnecessary; the limitation should be translated into a clear functional need, such as shorter hours, breaks, remote work, or a temporary change of tasks.

Significant difficulties are not always visible in a brief examination. Fatigue, pain, cognitive slowing, anxiety, and difficulty concentrating may become apparent only after a real attempt to return to routine. A further review point is therefore needed after several weeks and months, with the option to update goals and accommodations. Measures of success should include the person's ability to sustain a chosen role and sense of control, not merely a professional score measured in the treatment room.

This continuum requires connection among community medicine, rehabilitation professions, social services, and the setting to which the person returns. A coordinating professional should verify that a functional recommendation became a practical accommodation and that no gap emerged between formal entitlement and the ability to participate. Measures can include time to a gradual return, the proportion of accommodations implemented, persistence after six months, and the need to change course. Rehabilitation thus does not end at the door of the institute; it is tested where the person seeks to live life.

Checkpoints Along the Patient Journey

Stage	Information That Must Be Transferred	Responsible Owner	Completion Measure
Referral	Clinical question, urgency, and previous tests	Referring professional	The destination received and acknowledged the referral
Admission to the institution	Medications, allergies, and accessibility needs	Clinical receiving team	Verification with the patient or companion
Discharge	Changes in treatment and warning signs	Discharging department	Understanding and a scheduled follow-up appointment
Transition to community care	Summary, open results, and tasks	Coordinator or family physician	Closure of tasks within a defined timeframe
Digital channel	Notification together with a human alternative	Sending organization	No patient remains without access

Continuity is not a property of a discharge document but of a connection that has been completed. At every transition, it should be clear who hands off, who receives, and who verifies that information became action. When no one holds responsibility through to the end, the system may appear sound within every unit and still fail precisely in the space between them.

Chapter Eight: Violence in the Healthcare System - Development, Risk Factors, and the Human Cost

Opening Dilemma

A father waits with a child who is in pain. After two hours he is told that they will be seen soon; an hour later, another employee says that there is no way to estimate the time. He sees patients entering before them, raises his voice, and approaches the nurses' station. At first he is expressing anger; at the next stage, a sense of threat emerges. A professional response should set a clear boundary - threats or intimidating physical approach are unacceptable - while also providing reliable information, moving the conversation away from a crowded area, and checking whether the child's condition has changed. A time that cannot be met should not be promised, because a broken promise intensifies the sense of humiliation. The scenario shows that boundary-setting and listening can be combined.

There is no right to treatment within a space in which the caregiver fears for their life.

Violence against healthcare staff is a global, multifactorial phenomenon ranging from threats and humiliation to lethal assault; it harms workers, patients, and the system's ability to provide care.

1. Definition and Scope: Beyond the 'Exceptional Incident'

Violence in healthcare includes physical assault, threats, verbal abuse, sexual harassment, and damage to property. The normalization of verbal violence conceals both the scale of the phenomenon and its cumulative effects. For years, curses and threats were treated as part of the job, particularly in emergency departments, psychiatry, and geriatrics. Research and regulation increasingly framed them as an occupational hazard and a patient-safety problem (Ministry of Health, 2020; WHO, ILO, ICN & PSI, 2002).

When this principle is translated into practice, low reporting rates often reflect distrust, fear of being labeled, and a sense that nothing can be done. Without data, management has difficulty identifying recurring hours, locations, and patterns. A nurse who receives threats on every shift may not submit a report because no physical injury occurred. Over time, however, she may develop anxiety, burnout, and a desire to leave (WHO, ILO, ICN & PSI, 2002; Blumenthal et al., 2021).

The picture is not one-dimensional: not every aggressive behavior arises from the same degree of responsibility. Delirium, dementia, psychosis, or severe pain require an adapted clinical response, but they do not eliminate the duty to protect staff. Violent incidents in Israel have received public attention and led to initiatives involving security, penalties, and training. Yet the discussion often intensifies after a serious event and then fades.

A uniform definition, simple reporting, root-cause analysis, and post-incident support are foundational. Clinical management of behavior must be distinguished from enforcement against intentional violence.

2. Where and When Risk Increases

The risk of violence rises in settings marked by waiting, uncertainty, bad news, substance use, lack of privacy, and a feeling that no one is available to explain. Historically, emergency departments and psychiatric wards have been recognized worldwide as high-risk settings, but violence also occurs in clinics, ambulances, nursing homes, and home visits.

Within service delivery, environmental design matters: blocked exits, crowded rooms, unclear signage, and the absence of a safe conversation area increase stress. Staffing shortages may also leave a single employee facing an angry group. For example, a family that does not understand why others were taken in first may interpret clinical triage as discrimination. An information screen, proactive explanation, and periodic updates can reduce escalation.

At the same time, heavy security may deter violence but can also create a hostile atmosphere and harm populations that already fear institutions. The response should be tailored to the setting and level of risk. Israel's security environment adds sensitivity to the presence of guards and screening procedures. Teams also cope with mass-casualty emergencies and families under extreme stress.

Risk mapping, physical design, alarm systems, response teams, and proactive communication are preferable to relying solely on punishment after an event.

3. Workload, Waiting, and Uncertainty as Escalation Mechanisms

Workload does not justify violence, but it helps explain how accumulated frustration becomes confrontation. Identifying the mechanism is essential for prevention and does not assign blame to the victim. Historically, public systems have faced gaps between demand and capacity. When the public expects an immediate right but encounters a queue, the message can be experienced as a promise that has been broken.

In clinical reality, uncertainty is sometimes harder than the wait itself. A person who receives an estimated time and an update is more able to regulate anger than someone who does not know whether they have been forgotten. In an emergency department, prioritizing a life-threatening case over someone who arrived earlier can appear arbitrary. Explaining the triage method does not relieve pain, but it gives the process a logic.

Improved communication, however, is not a substitute for added resources. Using 'explanation' to mask a chronic shortage can transfer responsibility for a budgetary failure onto frontline workers. In Israel, hospital crowding, bed shortages, and periods of seasonal morbidity create conditions in which both staff and the public can reach the limits of their capacity. This is a foreseeable organizational risk.

Prevention combines shorter processes, flow management, flexible staffing, family updates, and an avenue for concerns before anger becomes a threat.

4. Effects of Violence on Staff and Quality of Care

Violence does not end when the incident ends; it changes professional behavior, harms concentration, deepens burnout, and increases turnover and feelings of alienation toward patients. Occupational-health studies have linked exposure to violence with psychological distress, absence from work, and intention to leave. The World Health Organization treats protection of workers as part of the core of a functioning health system (Myers-JDC-Brookdale Institute and Ministry of Health, 2023).

For the institution, an employee who has experienced an incident may avoid contact, shorten conversations, or practice defensive medicine. Violence against one worker can therefore harm subsequent patients as well. For example, a physician who was threatened after refusing an unjustified demand may comply the next time in order to avoid confrontation, even when that is not medically appropriate. Violence can alter clinical decision-making.

Nevertheless, support should not turn every worker into a helpless victim. Employees should be offered choices among conversation, therapy, leave, and legal assistance, while different coping styles are respected. In Israel, where many healthcare workers combine shifts, reserve duty, and heavy workloads, a violent incident is added to an already substantial burden. A rapid return to work without processing the event may look efficient but deepen the harm.

A post-incident procedure should include medical care, psychological support, debriefing, preservation of evidence, and assistance in dealing with the police. A manager should make contact rather than leave the employee to manage everything alone.

5. Between Enforcement and Systemic Prevention

Punishment is necessary in cases of intentional violence, but it is not sufficient. A safe system combines clear boundaries, planning, training, communication, and attention to workload-related drivers. Historically, public responses to severe incidents tend to focus on harsher penalties and more security guards. These steps signal a boundary, but the evidence on prevention supports a multilayered approach.

From an organizational perspective, a zero-tolerance policy should define a response rather than promise zero incidents. It can fail if employees do not know whom to contact or if management dismisses a complaint as 'part of the job.' A patient who curses because of a wait may receive a boundary and warning; a confused person requires clinical intervention; an intentional assailant requires removal and enforcement. The same response to all three is neither fair nor effective.

In practice, staff protection is not opposed to patients' rights. A violent environment harms privacy, availability, and the care of everyone. Conversely, disproportionate security force can harm dignity and trust. In Israel, public discourse can move from the slogan of a 'hard hand' toward a model of shared safety. Police, the Ministry of Health, employers, and workers' organizations should share information and responsibility.

A national program should include data, security standards, environmental planning, de-escalation training, legal response, and support, alongside investment in services that reduce predictable frustration.

A Prevention System: Violence in the Emergency Department

Violence in an emergency department does not begin at the moment of a threat. It develops within a physical space, a queue, changing messages, fatigue, and a gap between expectation and capacity. This section describes a prevention system that connects information, environmental design, de-escalation, security, and support for the employee after an incident.

An escalation pathway can often be identified early: frustration develops when a person does not know how long the wait will be, receives inconsistent answers, or sees others entering first without explanation. Early signs include repeated approaches, a rising voice, physical encroachment, and focused accusations. The team should recognize the sequence rather than wait for an explicit threat.

An early response combines a factual update, acknowledgment of difficulty, and a clear boundary. One staff member leads the conversation to avoid contradictory messages and, when possible, moves it to a quieter place. No commitment should be made unless it is supported by information; it is better to explain what is known, what remains unknown, and when another update will be given.

Security as Part of the Clinical System

A security officer is not a substitute for adequate staffing, but should be part of response planning. Familiarity with the emergency department layout, de-escalation training, and a clear link with the clinical lead allow security presence to reduce rather than intensify a threat. Police are required when there is an actual danger or an offense that cannot be managed through institutional measures.

Any use of force should be proportionate and documented, while necessary medical care continues. A behavioral boundary is not a denial of treatment: the presence of a companion may be limited, the location may be changed, or supervised access may be required, but such a decision must be explained and reviewed.

A Recovery Pathway for the Employee and the Team

After a violent incident, the safety review should be separated from support for the employee. The employee may need medical treatment, an opportunity to leave the shift, information about reporting, and psychological support that is not framed as weakness. A manager should make contact in the days after the event as well, because delayed reactions may include anxiety, avoidance, or a loss of professional confidence.

In parallel, a non-blaming debrief should ask what triggered the incident, which signs appeared, what worked, and what was missing. Conclusions should lead to a visible change - staffing adjustment, a change in messaging, physical redesign, or training - rather than ending with the event being entered into a reporting system.

What should be measured: counting assaults alone is insufficient. A prevention system also needs indicators that precede harm: near misses, threats that did not materialize, repeated calls to security, hours in which approaches to the staff desk accumulate, and times when staffing does not match workload. An increase in reporting after a campaign may indicate greater trust rather than worsening violence, so the number should be read alongside reporting rates, response times, post-incident absence, and employees' sense of safety. Data should return to the unit quickly and in a form that supports action: changing staffing deployment, correcting a message, opening a conversation area, or adapting security. Patient experience can also serve as an environmental indicator, not as a measure of 'dangerousness.' Repeated complaints about lack of information, unexplained waiting, or a threatening atmosphere may identify a friction point that can be corrected before it becomes an escalation. Breakdown by location, time, language, and service type is intended to identify working conditions and service patterns, not to label a group. Preventive measures should also be distinguished from their outcomes: training is measured by the team's ability to recognize signs and act together; a physical change is measured by whether friction is reduced, not merely displaced to another corridor; employee support is measured in part by a safe return to work. Another indicator is time to close the loop: when was the problem identified, who took responsibility, and what changed as a result? In this way, measurement serves the chapter as a practical safety system rather than as an argument over blame.

A follow-up plan after repeated incidents: when the same pattern of threat or confrontation recurs around ongoing treatment, each episode should not be handled as an isolated event. The organization should define who leads the conversation, which companions may participate, when a senior person is called, and what safety conditions apply to the next encounter. The plan should address concrete behavior and risk, not identity or diagnosis. When appropriate, a conversation or mediation may take place after the event, but no injured employee should be forced into such a meeting, and it should not replace necessary enforcement. The plan should be documented in a way accessible to relevant staff, limited to necessary information, and updated when circumstances change. After each significant encounter, the organization should check whether the arrangement worked and whether a new risk emerged. The goal is to prevent the same sequence, preserve continuity of care, and avoid leaving an employee to improvise alone.

De-escalation as a Team Skill

De-escalation is not a personality trait of a calm employee; it is a skill that can be practiced. It includes early recognition of tension, maintaining distance, using short sentences, avoiding humiliation, and offering limited choices. Equally important is knowing when to stop and call for help. Training should be based on scenarios from the actual department rather than a general lecture. Simulation allows the team to practice role allocation: who speaks, who calls for assistance, who moves other patients away, and who continues medical care. Language and culture affect interpretation of behavior. A loud voice, eye contact, or physical proximity may be understood differently. Risk signs should not be dismissed in the name of sensitivity, but cultural difference should not be converted automatically into a threat. An interpreter or mediator can prevent escalation when misunderstanding is central. Training should address bias and examine whether certain groups receive coercive responses more quickly. Data on security involvement and restraint by group can reveal a problem.

Violence Within Families and Between Patients

The emergency department must also address violence that is not directed at staff. A threatening partner, a family conflict, or a patient harming another person require protection and privacy. Staff should know how to separate people, identify domestic violence, and involve appropriate services. A sensitive conversation should not be conducted in the presence of a person suspected of causing harm. Environmental design and companion policies affect the ability to protect. When a minor or dependent person is involved, the duty to protect may require reporting. The decision should not be left to one employee under pressure. A rapid consultation pathway involving social work, a senior physician, and safeguarding services helps. Facts rather than assumptions should be documented, and the patient should be told, as far as possible, what is going to happen. Transparency can reduce the feeling that the system is acting behind the person's back, even when complete confidentiality cannot be preserved.

Physical and Pharmacological Restraint

Restraint is a serious intervention sometimes used for immediate protection. It should be a last resort, limited to what is necessary and for the shortest possible time. The reason, alternatives attempted, and reassessment should be documented. The team must monitor breathing, medical status, and dignity. After the event, it is appropriate to explain to the patient what was done and hear the patient's experience. Such a review may reveal whether earlier action could have prevented the restraint. A reduction in restraint rates is not sufficient if injuries are increasing. Safety for all parties must be examined. An institution can require review of every prolonged or repeated restraint and identify patterns by department and time. If the same person is repeatedly restrained, an individualized plan is needed. If restraint rates are high on a particular shift, training or staffing may be inadequate. In this way, information leads to targeted correction.

Environmental design to reduce friction: physical space influences behavior before any staff member speaks. A counter that is too low, a corridor without an exit, noise, harsh lighting, and lack of privacy increase tension. In contrast, clear sight lines, waiting areas organized by need, accessible signage, and a place for sensitive conversation help staff identify distress and respond early.

Safe design should not turn the emergency department into a fortress. Heavy barriers and threatening language can communicate suspicion toward everyone seeking care. Physical protection and accessibility must be balanced: a safe exit for employees, panic buttons, furniture that is difficult to throw, and a space that permits respectful proximity. Staff and patients should participate in planning because each group sees different blind spots.

After an environmental change, the institution should measure not only violent events but also repeated inquiries, perceived safety, and response time. If incidents simply move to another area, the improvement was only local.

Staff Fatigue and Mutual Escalation

A tired employee is more likely to shorten an explanation, interpret a question as disrespect, and respond sharply. A patient who is already in pain or uncertainty receives that message and intensifies the approach. A cycle then develops in which each side sees the other's response as proof of hostility. Violence prevention therefore requires attention to shifts, breaks, and rotation, not only communication training.

Teams can use proactive handoff: when a conversation becomes stuck, another staff member steps in without framing it as a failure. A short briefing at the start of a shift can identify patients in distress, but should avoid labels such as 'difficult' that harden negative expectations. It is better to describe the need and trigger: anxiety, prolonged waiting, or a language difficulty.

A manager who recognizes overload and permits a short break after an incident prevents accumulated strain from being carried into the next encounter. Worker safety and communication quality are two sides of the same working condition.

Non-Punitive Reporting: Employees avoid reporting when they fear being blamed for failing to prevent the event or when the form is long and produces no visible benefit. A credible system separates reporting for learning from disciplinary investigation in exceptional cases. It gives information back to the employee: what has been done, who is reviewing the event, and when an answer will be available.

Near misses and threats that did not materialize should also be reported because they expose conditions before injury occurs. At the same time, not every expression of patient anger should be classified as violence. Accurate classification protects the right to criticize and allows resources to be focused on dangerous situations.

A quarterly report to staff can present trends and corrective actions. When employees see that a change in staffing or signage resulted from their reports, willingness to participate increases.

Restoring Trust After an Incident

A violent incident also affects other patients who witness it. Some become afraid to approach staff, while others may learn that raising one's voice is the way to obtain attention. After a significant event, a general message can clarify that care is continuing, the team is safe, and concerns will be heard without violence. Details should not be disclosed, and the person involved should not be turned into a public example.

When safe and appropriate, a mediated meeting later may allow apology, explanation, and agreement on boundaries for continued care. Such a process is not appropriate after serious assault and does not replace enforcement, but in some conflicts it can prevent rupture and inadequate care. The employee must be protected from pressure to participate, and the patient must understand the conditions of the meeting.

Restoring trust is measured by the ability to continue treatment without erasing the harm. A system that responds only with exclusion or only with forgiveness does not provide a complete answer; boundary, accountability, and a safe path back to a therapeutic relationship are all required.

When the Threat Continues Outside the Hospital

A violent incident does not always end when the patient or companion leaves. Messages, photographing an employee, posting identifying details online, or waiting near the employee's car can extend the threat into the employee's home life. A procedure that addresses only what happened in the department leaves the worker alone at the point when fear becomes personal and persistent.

An organizational response should include preservation of evidence, risk assessment, assistance in contacting police when appropriate, protection of contact information, and guidance about social media. When identifying information has been posted, the organization should assist with removal requests rather than expect the employee to battle platforms alone. A shift change, escort to parking, or temporary work in another area may be protective measures, but they should not become a punishment that removes the harmed employee from work.

Management should clarify who communicates with the threatening person if medical care is still required. Sometimes one designated channel, clear boundaries, and security presence can be established; in other cases, care should be transferred to another team without abandoning the patient. The decision combines safety, continuity, and avoidance of further personal confrontation.

Follow-up should continue after the threat subsides. Sleep, absence, avoidance of particular shifts, and the team's sense of safety should be assessed. Brief support on the day of the incident is not enough when exposure continues online or when the employee fears the person will return. Closure should be based on the state of risk and the employee's condition, not on the moment the emergency-department door closed.

Violence Within the Team and Hierarchy That Prevents Reporting

Safety in healthcare is harmed not only by violence from patients and companions. Humiliation, threats, shouting, harassment, and bullying between employees can become a hidden routine, especially in hierarchical structures where junior staff depend on evaluations, shifts, and recommendations. Internal violence also affects patients: a team that is afraid to speak has difficulty warning about an error, asking for help, or stopping an unsafe action.

A sharp professional critique should be distinguished from an abusive pattern. Criticism addresses an action, allows a response, and aims at correction; bullying humiliates the person, recurs, isolates, or uses power to silence. Workload is not a justification, but it can increase risk, which means working conditions must be addressed as well as individual behavior.

A reporting pathway is not credible if a complaint automatically returns to the supervisor who is the subject of the complaint. An alternative address, confidential consultation, protection against retaliation, and a response timeframe are needed. At the same time, fair process must be protected for the person against whom an allegation is made. Review should focus on pattern, witnesses, messages, and impact, rather than simply asking who is more senior or who is perceived as more 'resilient.'

Organizational indicators can include psychological safety to raise concerns, staff transfers between units, absence, and repeated reports around the same focal point. Correction may require training, a management change, separation of reporting lines, or disciplinary action. Recognizing internal violence does not obscure the external threat; it completes the principle that people who protect patients are entitled to a safe work environment from colleagues as well.

Response Continuum for Escalation in the Emergency Department

Stage	**Early Sign**	**System Response**	**What Is Documented**
Waiting	Uncertainty and repeated inquiries	Proactive update and a timeframe	Duration of waiting and messages provided
Frustration	Rising voice, accusations, and physical encroachment	One staff member leads; conversation in an appropriate place	Trigger and calming steps
Threat	Explicit statement or dangerous gesture	Clear boundary and proportionate call for assistance	Level of threat and response
Active incident	Injury or attempted injury	Protection, separation, and medical care	Harm, witnesses, and use of force
After the incident	Anxiety, avoidance, or anger within the	Support, debriefing, and change of	Employee follow-up and corrective

Stage	Early Sign	System Response	What Is Documented
	team	conditions	actions

A good safety program does not measure only how many assailants were removed. It asks whether the team received information, whether waiting was managed, whether there was someone to call, and whether the harmed employee received continuing support. Responsibility for setting a boundary remains clear, but it is distributed among environmental design, staffing, management, and enforcement. From here, the discussion turns to a different question: not how to prevent violence in practice, but whether a change in its extent can be attributed to the discourse of patients' rights itself. That is the question of Chapter Nine.

Chapter Nine: Causal Relationship or Coincidental Correlation? Patients' Rights, Authority, and Violence

Opening Dilemma

A researcher compares three departments over five years before and after the introduction of a rights-based procedure. Incidents are collected by severity, waiting time, workload, and changes in reporting, while employees and patients are interviewed in parallel. If verbal complaints increase but assaults decrease, the finding does not support a simple story of escalation. The conflict may have moved into an institutional channel. Even a strong design has limitations: departments change, staff turn over, and rare events create uncertainty. The report should present alternatives and avoid a causal headline. Its value lies in identifying a mechanism and testing an intervention, not in declaring that a complex social issue has been solved by a single number. Causal analysis matters because it influences solutions. The example below does not describe a study conducted for this book; it illustrates how the claim could be examined systematically and cautiously.

When two phenomena rise together, we still do not know which caused the other - or whether both were driven by a third force.

There is insufficient basis for concluding that the Patients' Rights Law caused an increase in violence. Rights discourse and consumerism may have changed expectations, but any effect is mediated by workload, inequality, communication, culture, and enforcement capacity.

1. How to Examine a Causal Claim

The claim that the law created violence requires more than temporal proximity. One must show a mechanism, a measurable change, a comparison, and a reasonable exclusion of alternative explanations. Historically, the 1996 law was enacted during a period in which society was also changing in communication, consumerism, inequality, and attitudes toward authority. Reporting of violence also improved, so an increase in reported incidents does not necessarily mean an equivalent increase in actual events.

When the principle meets the system, causality can be examined by comparing sectors, periods, and countries; testing whether knowledge of rights predicts violence; and examining processes within individual events. Such analysis is complex and vulnerable to bias. For example, if a patient says 'it is my right' during a threat, that statement does not prove that the law caused the behavior. The term may be used as a justification after anger arose because of waiting or refusal.

At the same time, absence of proof is not proof of no effect. Rights discourse may shape expectations indirectly. Conclusions should therefore be expressed in degrees of certainty rather than as a complete acquittal or conviction. In Israel, a serious examination of the issue should connect police data, institutional reports, employee surveys, and patient experience. At present, different sources use different definitions and periods.

Before changing the law, the mechanism should be examined. A solution that weakens rights without evidence may harm patients and fail to reduce violence. It is preferable to intervene in established risk factors.

2. The Hypothesis of Eroding Professional Authority

Patient empowerment challenged unilateral authority, but it was not meant to abolish professional authority. The problem arises when partnership is interpreted as an obligation to satisfy every demand. The transition from paternalism to autonomy occurred alongside a broader decline in trust in experts. The internet and social media expanded access to information but also spread misinformation and presented opinion as if it were an equal alternative to evidence.

From an institutional perspective, when an organization markets choice and service without explaining limits, frontline staff are left to say 'no' to a marketing promise. The contradiction weakens their position. A patient who arrives with a self-diagnosis and demands treatment may perceive refusal as arrogance. The physician can respond dismissively or turn the encounter into a shared examination of information, risk, and alternatives.

Professional authority, however, is not immunity from criticism. It is legitimate when grounded in knowledge, transparent, humble, and open to challenge. Authority that demands obedience solely because of a title invites resistance. In Israel, direct communication may be understood as assertiveness or as disrespect. Training in communication and boundary-setting allows staff to preserve professionalism without being drawn into a status struggle.

The public should be told both rights and limits: a right to explanation and a second opinion, not a right to compel treatment that lacks an indication; a right to dignity, alongside a duty to avoid violence and consider others.

3. 'I Am Entitled to It,' Consumerism, and Unlimited Expectations

Aggressive entitlement may grow from a combination of rights language and market language, but asserting a right should not itself be equated with violence or selfishness. Historically, public discourse shifted from the passive service recipient to the consumer who compares, rates, and threatens to change providers. In healthcare, some services are publicly funded and others purchased, which blurs the boundaries.

Within service structures, systems invite feedback but sometimes reward managers solely on satisfaction scores. Employees may feel that the organization will side with the complainant at any cost, even when that person harms them. For example, a demand to bring a companion into a restricted area may reflect a genuine need or disregard for the privacy of others. A solution requires explanation, consistent exceptions, and an avenue of appeal - not a power struggle.

Yet the phrase 'I am entitled to it' can also express historical correction. Groups that were previously excluded sometimes need to be forceful to obtain basic service. The assertiveness of a weaker party should not automatically be labeled as a threat. In Israel, personal connections and 'protektzia' alongside formal rights can create a sense that those who do not push will be left behind. This encourages competitive behavior around a public resource.

Equal procedures, transparent waiting times, and credible appeals reduce the need to shout as a strategy. The organization should demonstrate that lawful pathways work and that violence does not shorten the queue.

4. Structural Explanations as a Test of the Causal Account

Chapter Eight presented shortages, waiting, uncertainty, substance use, and social tension as practical risk factors for escalation. In this chapter they play a different role: they are confounding variables that must be considered before changes in violence are attributed to rights discourse. If workload, staffing, or reporting patterns changed during the same period, temporal proximity to a law or rights procedure is not enough to establish causality.

Causally, the source of frustration should be separated from the language in which it is expressed. A patient may use the term 'right' during a confrontation, but the confrontation may have originated in waiting, scarcity, or an organizational decision that the frontline employee has no authority to change. Coding words spoken during an incident is therefore not equivalent to identifying the cause that generated it.

Comparisons among institutions, periods, and countries can help. If violence also appears in systems where rights discourse is very different, and if it clusters particularly around workload and uncertainty, the need for a multifactorial explanation becomes stronger. Even then, responsibility is not removed from the person who commits violence; the distinction is intended to determine what explains the trend and what merely accompanies it.

Staffing, patient flow, waiting times, information, accessibility, enforcement, and changes in reporting should therefore be included in the analytic model. Only after accounting for them can one ask whether rights discourse retains an independent and meaningful explanatory contribution.

5. An Integrated Model: Rights with Mutual Responsibility

The way forward is not retreat from rights but a move from one-sided rights toward an institutional compact that defines rights, boundaries, and responsibilities of patients, staff, and the state. Documents such as the NHS Constitution combine rights of patients and employees with public responsibilities. The model does not deny a right; it recognizes that a shared system requires reciprocal conduct.

In practical terms, patients are entitled to information, dignity, and appropriate care; workers are entitled to safety, dignity, and institutional backing; and the state is responsible for resources and rules. The balance cannot be placed solely on the encounter at the counter. For example, when a request is denied, the patient receives an explanation and a route of appeal; when the patient threatens, the organization sets a boundary and supports the worker; when a delay results from shortage, management does not hide behind frontline staff.

However, responsibility discourse can be used to blame patients or make treatment conditional on behavior. Urgent treatment is not a reward, and worker protection should be proportionate and non-discriminatory. In Israel, patients' rights discourse could be updated through a complementary charter on rights and safety in healthcare without reducing existing legal protections.

Separate hypotheses should therefore be tested: changes in expectations, the effect of appeals, the role of workload, and institutional boundaries. Breaking the issue into mechanisms is more precise than a single measure of 'violence.'

A Framework for Systematically Examining the Relationship Between Rights and Violence

To avoid anecdotal conclusions, the examination should distinguish among incident types, measure actual exposure to rights discourse, and compare alternative explanations over time. The framework below does not propose another violence-prevention program - Chapter Eight addressed that task - but defines the data and analytical steps required to test whether there is an independent causal relationship.

A common language for incidents: monitoring begins with definitions that do not confuse criticism with violence. Complaint, argument, insult, threat, harassment, property damage, and physical assault should be distinguished, while severity and the identity of the harmed party are recorded. Uniform classification permits comparison among institutions without encouraging over-reporting or concealment.

Alongside incident type, it is important to record whether care was disrupted, an employee was absent from work, or force was used. The data then reflect not only the number of events but also their organizational and human cost.

Linking the incident to the service context: an isolated event does not explain itself. It should be linked to waiting time, occupancy, staffing shortages, shift changes, messages communicated to the patient, and characteristics of the location. This connection does not assign blame to the system or the patient; it makes it possible to identify which conditions repeatedly precede escalation.

Context data should be collected automatically where possible so that reporting does not burden the employee. The system can draw admission times, workload, and staffing levels automatically, while the employee adds a short description of the trigger and response.

Sentinel Sites and a National Sample

Instead of requiring every institution to operate a complete system from the first day, implementation can begin with sentinel sites representing emergency departments, community clinics, mental-health services, and geriatric institutions. These sites would collect detailed data and test the reliability of definitions. In parallel, a reduced dataset would be collected across the entire system.

After a pilot period, components that proved useful can be expanded and fields that do not contribute to understanding can be removed. Monitoring is then built through learning rather than through a long form that is difficult to maintain.

Privacy and Data Governance

Violence reports contain sensitive information about patients and employees. An operational database used to manage individual cases should be separated from a de-identified research database. Access to identifiable information should be limited to clearly defined roles, and every secondary use should require approval and oversight.

A joint data-governance committee including the Ministry of Health, workers' organizations, patient representatives, and privacy experts should define retention periods, permissions, and publication rules. Broad representation helps prevent the database from being used for punishment or broad labeling of groups.

Coding Institutional Messages and Actual Exposure

The term 'rights discourse' is not a single variable. What was actually presented should be documented: signage, intake materials, public campaigns, employee training, wording of notices, and the functioning of appeal channels. Two institutions subject to the same law may communicate very different messages - one emphasizes partnership and fairness, while another presents a list of entitlements without boundaries or a practical pathway.

An exposure index is therefore needed rather than reliance on an official date: how many patients saw the message, what they understood from it, whether employees used it in conversation, and whether a credible appeal pathway was opened. Only then should exposure be connected to other outcomes. Measurement does not itself prove causation; its purpose is to ensure that the analysis is examining a real intervention rather than attributing influence to a document no one read.

Reconstructing the Event Sequence from Multiple Sources

For a selected case, an integrated timeline should be built from admission records, waiting times, security calls, clinical documentation, messages sent, and accounts from the parties involved. Each source sees a different part; an employee's account does not cancel the patient's experience, and vice versa. The discrepancies themselves may point to a message that was misunderstood, a change that was not documented, or a decision for which no one held clear authority.

The reconstruction is not a disciplinary process and does not by itself determine legal responsibility. It searches for the turning point: when frustration became a threat, what option was available at that moment, and what prevented its use. The conclusion should be a testable action - a change in messaging, manager availability, queue design, or employee protection - rather than a general statement about 'poor communication.'

Dashboard and Early Warning: An institutional dashboard should present trends, not names: incident rates by unit, waiting times, absence after injury, and use of restraint. A persistent deviation should trigger review rather than automatic sanction. Sometimes increased reporting indicates greater confidence in the reporting system.

An early-warning system can identify combinations of overload, turnover, and repeated incidents and trigger staffing reinforcement, communication changes, or environmental adaptation. Human judgment remains essential to avoid inappropriate labeling.

A Public Report That Presents Complexity: An annual report should publish definitions, reporting rates, differences among settings, and corrective actions. A competitive table ranking the 'most violent institution' should not be published without adjustment for activity volume and patient population, because such ranking may encourage concealment.

The report should also present limitations, changes in measurement methods, and examples of interventions that succeeded or failed. This kind of transparency supports public discussion that does not automatically blame patients or staff.

Staggered Design and Comparison Between Units

A staggered evaluation can begin in a number of diverse institutions where the timing and nature of changes in rights presentation, appeal channels, or service messages are known. Rather than relying on a simple 'before and after' comparison, similar units in which the change occurred at a different time should be included to test whether the trend changes around actual exposure.

The exposure point, primary outcome, and reasonable time window for change should be specified in advance. A change that began months before the intervention, or appears equally in comparison units, weakens the causal claim. This reduces post hoc interpretation tailored to the observed result.

An independent evaluation should also assess fidelity of exposure: did the new message actually reach patients and employees, was it understood similarly, and did other changes occur at the same time in staffing, security, or reporting? Without this check, one cannot know whether the result reflects rights discourse or another concurrent change.

Data Quality and Bias Control

A monitoring system can create an illusion of precision. A unit that reports more may appear more dangerous even if its culture is more open, while a unit that conceals events may appear safer. Reporting completion rates, time from incident to report, and discrepancies among employee reports, security records, and patient complaints should therefore be measured. Such cross-checking does not eliminate bias, but it makes it visible.

The organization should periodically test whether two reporters classify the same description at the same severity level. Low agreement means that definitions or training are insufficient. Sample audits of records, security calls, and absences can uncover events that never entered the database.

Changes in the reporting system should be clearly marked in the time series. Otherwise, an increase caused by a new form may be interpreted as worsening reality. A data-quality report should be published alongside the findings, not hidden in a footnote.

Time-Series Analysis and Staggered Changes

To identify a trend, months and years should be examined rather than two points in time. A time series can reveal seasonality, winter workload, staffing changes, or an exceptional public event. When an intervention is implemented, the analysis can test for a change in the level or slope of the series and compare it with similar units that did not implement the intervention at the same time.

Such comparison is not a randomized trial, but it is stronger than a simple before-and-after impression. The intervention date and primary outcome should be defined in advance, and the analysis should test whether the change had already begun. If a unit was selected for a pilot precisely because its situation was extreme, some improvement may reflect natural regression to the mean.

Proper analysis should present uncertainty intervals and sensitivity to different definitions. The goal is a reasonable decision, not a single sharp number that hides its limitations.

Primary Outcomes, Secondary Outcomes, and Unintended Harms

A single outcome is insufficient for causal assessment. Alongside incident rates, complaint, threat, and assault should be distinguished, and severity, injuries, absences, security use, and patient complaints should also be examined. Increased reporting alongside fewer assaults may represent a healthier reporting culture rather than worsening violence.

The primary outcome and secondary outcomes should be specified in advance so that the measure supporting the preferred claim is not chosen afterward. If exposure to rights discourse was partial or inconsistent, absence of change does not prove absence of effect; it may show that the measured intervention barely occurred.

The analysis should also examine different groups. A system-wide average may conceal different patterns among people who do not speak Hebrew, people with disabilities, mental-health settings, or units where compulsory decisions are more common.

Resources as an Explanatory Variable: Changes in budget, staffing, occupancy, security, or service availability are not merely managerial matters; they can change violence levels independently of rights discourse. Resource data should therefore be included in the time series and comparative analysis.

For example, a decline in events after guards were added or a shift was reinforced cannot automatically be attributed to a new patient message. Likewise, staffing cuts may generate an increase that is mistakenly attributed to a 'demanding culture.'

The causal report should present these changes explicitly and test the sensitivity of the conclusion to their inclusion. The more the relationship between rights and violence disappears after adjustment for workload and resources, the weaker the claim of an independent effect becomes.

Shared Interpretation Without Turning Testimony into Causal Proof

After quantitative and case-level analysis, a small forum of employees, patient representatives, security staff, and managers can be convened to interpret the finding and select an intervention. The forum's role is not to collect testimony again, but to assess whether the explanation derived from the data is plausible to those who experience the service and work, and what possible cost the proposed solution may carry.

The forum should receive anonymized material and a clearly defined open question. When disagreement remains, the report should present more than one interpretation rather than determine by vote who is 'to blame.' A recommendation should be adopted only when it is clear who has authority to implement it, what will be measured, and what will count as an unintended harm - for example, shifting workload to another department or harming accessibility.

The combination of professional expertise and user experience serves here as a tool for critical interpretation, not a substitute for comparison and measurement. It helps ensure that a statistical model does not appear precise while remaining disconnected from how the service actually operates.

Denominator, Exposure, and Clustering of Events

Raw counts do not permit comparison among units. A department handling thousands of visits, operating around the clock, and receiving complex cases is expected to accumulate more incidents than a small clinic even if the risk per encounter is lower. Rates should therefore be presented relative to visits, inpatient days, operating hours, or staff-hours, depending on the setting.

The denominator should also reflect actual exposure. Extreme workload during specific two-hour windows, high turnover, or frequent compulsory decisions can create risk that is invisible in a daily average. Analysis by hour, location, and encounter type can identify a recurring window requiring redesign rather than attributing the problem to an entire population or one employee.

It is important to distinguish broad dispersion from repeated clustering. Dozens of minor incidents in different places require a different response from a series concentrated at the same reception point, cancellation process, or transfer between units. Anonymous linkage among incidents can reveal an operational pattern without creating a blacklist of patients or workers.

A responsible report should present the total count, the rate relative to exposure, and the degree of clustering in time and place together. When the denominator changes - for example because a service closes, operating hours change, or staffing falls - this should be stated explicitly. This allows distinction between an increase caused by more activity and a genuine change in risk per encounter.

Frequency, Severity, and Harm Are Not the Same Measure: Ten verbal confrontations and one physical assault cannot be combined into a single number without losing meaning. Frequency describes how often an event occurred; severity describes the type of injury or threat; harm includes absence from work, medical treatment, changes in staff behavior, and effects on other patients. A policy may reduce severe assaults even if the number of arguments remains similar.

A basket of outcomes is therefore required: incidents by severity level, injuries, downtime, security use, disruption of continuity, and perceived safety. Examining the distribution prevents a small change in minor incidents from hiding a rare but dangerous increase. It also permits a targeted intervention - such as a panic button - to be evaluated by the outcome it is actually meant to affect.

Separating the measures is especially important in causal debate. More demanding discourse may increase complaints or verbal confrontations without increasing physical violence; extreme workload or access to weapons may affect the severity of events instead. A graded conclusion is more accurate than a general declaration that violence rose or fell.

The Ethical Boundary of Experimenting with Rights Discourse

To test whether rights discourse affects violence, one might be tempted to assign departments different messages and measure incidents. But an organizational experiment cannot deny information, complaint mechanisms, or respectful treatment merely to create a control group. Basic rights are a condition of the study, not a variable that can be removed.

Different implementation methods can be compared so long as none falls below the mandatory standard: written messaging versus oral explanation, different frequencies of waiting-time updates, or the addition of a service mediator. Outcomes should include not only violence but also understanding, trust, privacy harm, and staff workload. An intervention that reduces reporting by silencing people is not a success.

Consent for organizational research also requires thought. An individual patient cannot always choose whether an entire corridor operates under a new procedure, but the experiment can be publicized, data collection minimized, objection to

secondary use of personal information enabled where appropriate, and public representatives involved in oversight. Employees need similar protection against their reports being used for disciplinary evaluation.

An ethics committee should assess the balance between expected knowledge and social risk. The causal investigation should not recreate the very concern it seeks to examine by producing a less respectful environment. The method remains rigorous, but its limits are defined by the same rights-based approach the book seeks to protect.

Minimum Requirements for a Cautious Causal Assessment

A good evaluation may reach a complex conclusion: rights discourse changes expectations but does not by itself explain violence; workload matters but does not remove personal responsibility. The practical advantage of a graded conclusion is that each mechanism can be addressed with the appropriate tool, rather than choosing between blaming patients and denying risk to staff.

Component	**Operational Question**	**Primary Risk**	**Required Safeguard**
Incident classification	What occurred and at what severity?	Mixing complaints with violence	Uniform glossary and training
Context data	Under what conditions did the event occur?	Drawing conclusions without workload and time	Automatic linkage to service data
Privacy	Who may view identifiable information?	Labeling a patient or employee	Separation of operational and research databases
Publication	What can be compared publicly?	Misleading ranking and concealment of reports	Adjustment for activity volume and presentation of limitations
Action	How does the data lead to correction?	Collection without change	Review threshold, accountable owner, and follow-up date

Part Four: A Cross-Continental Comparative View - Between Constitutional Declaration and Service in Practice

Comparison between countries is not a simple competition in ranking rights. A broad constitutional document may coexist with severe shortages, while a system without an explicit constitutional right may still provide universal service. The following chapters compare systems along four axes: the source of the right, financing structure, rights in the clinical encounter, and enforceability. Each chapter also asks what Israel can learn - and what cannot be imported because of historical, cultural, and institutional differences.

Why These Comparative Cases Were Chosen

The countries do not represent entire continents and are not ranked from best to worst. Each was selected because it highlights a different mechanism through which a right can be realized - or remain a declaration.

Comparative Case	Feature Examined	Central Tension	Possible Lesson for Israel
Brazil	Constitutional right and a universal public system	Regional disparities and financing alongside a broad promise	Link the anchoring of rights to budgetary responsibility and public participation.
Bolivia	Plurinational system and intercultural health	Respect for tradition versus individual liberty	Expand translation, mediation, and accommodation without giving up individual consent.
United States	Legal autonomy and a fragmented insurance system	Rights in the encounter without universal coverage	Distinguish formal freedom of choice from the economic ability to obtain care.
Canada	Broad public coverage and	Universality alongside waiting	Combine transparency about

Comparative Case	Feature Examined	Central Tension	Possible Lesson for Israel
	provincial management	times	availability with an alternative pathway in high-risk situations.
China	Expanded coverage, large hospitals, and digitalization	Workload, incentives, and trust	Connect rights with stronger primary care and transparency of information.
Japan	Universal insurance and broad access to providers	Overuse, ageing, and coordination	Develop continuity and workforce planning alongside broad freedom of access.
Thailand	Universal coverage and a no-fault assistance mechanism	Early compensation versus professional accountability	Consider a rapid corrective mechanism that does not replace investigation of failure.
Malaysia	Public-private system in a multi-religious society	Variation between institutions and end-of-life tensions	Set a clear national floor with cultural accommodation.
Nigeria	Federalism, an informal labor market, and expanding insurance	Fragmented responsibility and out-of-pocket payment	Publish the chain of responsibility and measure where the pathway breaks down.
South Africa	Constitutional right and progressive realization	Deep shortages and substantive equality	Connect priority-setting with reasons and review.
United Kingdom	National service and an accessible service constitution	Service promises versus waiting and workforce constraints	Bring rights and responsibilities together in an accessible public document that can be measured.
Germany	Compulsory insurance and professional self-governance	Institutional expertise versus complexity and legitimacy	Combine professional expertise, public representation, and transparency in benefit-package and quality decisions.

Chapter Ten: Latin America - Brazil and Bolivia

Opening Dilemma

A pregnant woman in a village in Bolivia is afraid to go to a hospital where she does not speak the language. A community worker and a traditional midwife help plan the referral, and the center commits to providing an interpreter and allowing a companion. When a risk sign appears, the woman arrives early. The right was realized not by a legal clause alone, but through connection, transportation, and accommodation. The same principle operates in Brazil when a family-health team identifies a person who is not attending follow-up. The local visit is not surveillance of the citizen, but a way to identify a barrier and offer a service. Privacy and consent remain protected, and the community does not become an arm of coercion. The Latin American experience also highlights the connection between social rights and democracy.

A constitutional declaration can open a gate; it does not by itself build the road leading to it.

Brazil and Bolivia anchor the right to health in strong public and constitutional language, but realization of that right is shaped by inequality, geography, resources, and tensions between Western models and community and Indigenous medicine.

1. The Right to Health in Latin America

The transition from dictatorships to democracies and the struggle against inequality turned health into a constitutional arena of citizenship, participation, and social justice. Historically, in the late twentieth century, countries in the region adopted new constitutions and a broad language of social rights. Community-health movements and professionals connected illness with poverty, land, race, and exclusion.

At the system level, constitutional anchoring enables judicial review and requires the state to justify policy. It can also generate litigation pressure when budgets and service capacity do not match the promise. A court order for an expensive medicine may save an individual life, but if it bypasses priority-setting it may shift resources from prevention and basic services toward those who are able to litigate.

Individual rights and collective justice, however, are not always identical. Rights adjudication should also ask who never reaches court and what the remedy costs others. Israel is similar in having strong judicial review, but differs in the absence of an explicit constitutional right to health. Health legislation fills part of that gap.

The lesson is to connect rights with a transparent budgetary process, public participation, and evidence. Courts are gatekeepers, not substitutes for health-system planning.

2. Brazil: The 1988 Constitution and SUS

Key sources: Constitution of Brazil, 1988, arts. 196-200.

Brazil declared health a right of all and a duty of the state and created the Sistema Unico de Saude (SUS) as a universal system based on comprehensiveness, decentralization, and social participation. Historically, the democratic Constitution of 1988 emerged after military rule and was influenced by the sanitary reform movement. Articles 196-200 linked health to social and economic policy and to reduction of risk.

In practice, SUS provides primary care, vaccination, emergency services, and complex care, and operates health councils and conferences for public participation. A substantial private sector exists alongside it. The Family Health Strategy, for example, represents an effort to bring teams into the community rather than wait for patients to reach hospitals. It connects prevention, home visits, and population mapping.

On the other hand, regional disparities, insufficient financing, and dependence on local authorities create variation. Legal universality does not guarantee equal availability in the Amazon and in a major city. Israel can learn from institutionalized public participation and from treating prevention as part of the right. Conversely, Israel's health funds provide organizational continuity that is difficult to reproduce in a broad federal model.

Anchoring rights should include stable financing, responsibility across levels of government, and public forums with real influence. Without these, the declaration remains vulnerable to the political cycle.

3. Bolivia: Universality, Plurinationalism, and Intercultural Health

Bolivia seeks to combine a universal right to health with recognition of Indigenous peoples and traditional medicine, and therefore challenges a uniform model of caregiver, knowledge, and consent. The 2009 Constitution defined the state as plurinational and strengthened social rights. The unified system was expanded to cover people not insured through social security.

What Intercultural Health Looks Like in the Encounter Itself

Intercultural accommodation is not limited to literal translation or displaying a community symbol. It begins by asking how the person explains the illness, which family members or traditional healers they wish to involve, and what might cause them to avoid the service. The team is not required to accept every explanation as medical evidence, but it should explain its recommendation without dismissing the patient's world. Where appropriate, clinical care and traditional support can be coordinated as long as risk, boundaries of responsibility, and the person's preference are clear.

A community mediator can open a door, but must not become the individual's exclusive spokesperson. A private conversation must also be possible, especially where there are power differences within the family or community. Success is measured not by the number of cultural encounters held, but by how many people complete treatment with understanding, by reduced avoidance, and by the ability to refuse without losing access to service. In this way, intercultural health protects both community belonging and personal liberty.

At the organizational level, the Salud Familiar Comunitaria Intercultural policy seeks to integrate community, family, and culture. The inclusion of traditional midwives is an example of recognition of local knowledge. A woman from an Indigenous community may prefer a particular birthing position, companion, or ritual not customary in a hospital. Safe accommodation can increase trust and access without abandoning clinical standards.

In implementation, cultural recognition is not beyond criticism. The individual's wishes, especially those of women and minors, must be protected even when community leadership presents a position in the name of tradition. Israel also includes communities with different understandings of family, modesty, and authority. The Bolivian model emphasizes community participation, but individual human rights within the group must remain protected.

Intercultural training, translation, mediation, and integration of community-based caregivers can improve accessibility. Accommodation should be based on consent, not stereotype.

4. The Right in the Constitution Versus Service in Practice

The gap between norm and reality in Latin America shows that the right to health depends on infrastructure, workforce, taxation, and state capacity no less than on constitutional wording. Historically, economic crises, political instability, and longstanding inequality disrupted continuity of reform. Epidemics exposed both the strengths of public systems and their shortages.

Within institutional design, decentralization can adapt services to local needs but deepen disparities when tax bases differ. Private financing can fill gaps while drawing personnel and resources away from the public system. A community clinic without medicines or staff, for example, does not realize a right even if care is formally free. The person must travel, pay, or forgo care.

This does not mean that constitutional declaration is worthless. It provides a language for organization, budgeting, and review. The question is how to translate it into measurable and progressive duties. Israel's infrastructure gap is smaller, but gaps remain in waiting times, the periphery, and the share of private financing. The comparison warns against relying on law without budgetary monitoring.

Multi-year targets, data by region and group, a core of services, and protection against regression are required. Progressive realization must be measurable.

5. Lessons for Israel: Participation, Community, and Justice

The central lesson from Latin America is that the right to health is not only a relationship between an individual and a physician, but a democratic project of participation, prevention, and reduction of disparities. Historically, health movements in the region viewed the community as a partner in defining needs. This differs from a model in which experts decide and the public is invited to comment afterward.

In practice, public councils can connect data with local experience, but they need authority, resources, and representation of groups that are not organized. Planning a peripheral clinic together with residents may reveal transportation, work-hour, and language barriers that were absent from a professional report.

Participation is nonetheless complex: it is not a referendum on every clinical decision. It is appropriate for priority-setting, service design, and evaluation of experience while professional standards remain intact. Israel could strengthen regional health councils, include patients on quality committees, and use disparity-adjusted financing. The health-fund structure permits broad pilots.

Participation should be early, diverse, and documented. The public should be shown how its input affected decisions; otherwise participation becomes a ritual without trust.

Policy and Community: Constitutional Right and Resource Allocation

Broad constitutional anchoring creates expectations, but realization depends on how budgets, workforce, distance, and culture are translated into services. This section examines mechanisms that connect a social right with district-level decisions, community participation, and oversight of resource allocation.

A social right is not a promise of everything - but it requires a pathway. It permits examination of whether priorities are reasonable, whether particular groups are being left behind, and whether the state is progressing rather than regressing. It does not mean every new service must be provided immediately, but shortage is not an exemption from giving reasons. When basic treatment is unavailable, the state should show the gap, how resources were allocated, and the improvement plan. A right without a timetable, budget, and measure can become a promise that is always postponed. Conversely, a demand for immediate provision of every treatment may bypass public priority-setting and harm broad services. Brazil's SUS distributes responsibility among federal, state, and local levels. Decentralization allows adaptation to need, but creates variation: a strong local authority may manage teams, data, and procurement more effectively than a poor one.

Local authority should therefore come with funding, professional support, and a national standard. A municipality cannot be made responsible for health without the ability to employ professionals or purchase medicines. At the same time, purely centralized management may miss distance, language, and needs that are invisible from the capital. The balance is a national floor with local choice about how to reach it. Community health councils in Brazil express the idea that the public is not merely a service recipient. They can expose shortages, scrutinize budgets, and change priorities. Yet participation does not occur merely because people are invited to a meeting. Information must be understandable, weaker areas must be represented, and people must have time to influence decisions before they are made. If councils are populated mainly by those who already have connections, they may reproduce disparities. The public role is to add knowledge and legitimacy, not to assume the state's responsibility for financing.

Litigation over Medicines and Its Budgetary Consequences

A legal proceeding may save a person who was denied a medicine, but large numbers of individual orders can shift resources toward those who are able to reach court. Alongside immediate relief, a public mechanism is therefore needed to publish criteria, assess costs and benefits, and provide a rapid appeal route for all patients.

Courts can require the state to use a transparent decision-making process rather than replace priority-setting themselves. In this way, an individual success can correct the mechanism instead of remaining an exception that deepens inequality.

Intercultural Medicine as a Safe Referral Pathway

Integrating traditional knowledge is not achieved simply by placing a cultural symbol in a clinic. It is necessary to define when a traditional healer may accompany a patient, how information is transferred, and which danger signs require rapid referral to medical care. Mutual recognition of roles reduces suspicion and prevents dangerous delay.

The test is whether patients can choose without being punished and without receiving promises that lack a basis. Documentation of referral, transportation availability, and community feedback turn cultural sensitivity into a safety mechanism rather than a romanticization of shortage.

Distance, workforce, and the meaning of availability: a clinic is not accessible merely because it appears on a map. If it is unstaffed, if medicine is unavailable, or if reaching it requires a full day of travel, the right remains formal. Access assessment should include travel time, operating hours, stock, professional availability, and out-of-pocket spending. Indirect costs should also be measured: lost workdays, childcare, and dependence on a companion. A national average number of facilities can conceal a region in which service is unavailable when needed. Recruiting and retaining personnel in peripheral areas require more than a one-time grant. Professionals need training, housing, professional support, advancement opportunities, and security. Telemedicine can shorten distance, but is not suitable for every examination and is inaccessible without infrastructure. A combination of a local team, remote consultation, and a defined referral pathway can create continuity, provided the patient is not required to mediate among levels of care alone.

How to measure progressive realization: progress in a social right should be measured over time and by subgroup. Possible indicators include functioning primary care, medication availability, workforce, travel time, out-of-pocket spending, and completion of referrals. A target of increasing the number of clinics is not useful if operating hours are shrinking. Community testimony is also needed alongside data because it reveals trust barriers and procedures that do not appear in databases. Transparent budgeting is part of the right. The public should know how much was allocated, which gap the budget was intended to reduce, and what happened in practice. Transparency is not a table alone; it requires an understandable explanation and an ability to ask questions. A community council may identify that a budget was consumed by inappropriate procurement or that a clinic was built in an inaccessible location. Responsibility for correction nonetheless remains with the competent authority. Participation is not a way to transfer failure to the community. To avoid symbolic participation, councils should receive data and have influence before decisions on hours, closure of services, or changes in pathways. At the same time, a strong local authority should not receive better service merely because it knows how to demand it. Compensatory financing and a national floor are conditions of fair decentralization.

Brazil: Public Participation Between Law and Reality

Their strength depends on information, representation, and the ability to influence budgets. If discussion takes place in technical language or at inaccessible times, the same people will return again and again. Support for participation - translation, transportation, and understandable data - is part of health democracy. What was decided and what was rejected should be published. Participation then becomes a mechanism of accountability rather than a ritual. Compensatory federal financing, professional assistance, and national standards are needed to guarantee a floor. Measurement should distinguish local capacity from local choice. When an authority cannot provide basic service, the state cannot simply say that responsibility was devolved. Public responsibility continues even when delivery is decentralized.

Shortage and the importance of reliable service: inventory management, procurement, and transportation are rights mechanisms. Information about shortages should be visible and include an alternative and estimated timeframe. When a person travels from far away and discovers that care is unavailable, the cost is not only financial. A system can use a call center, message, or community contact to prevent unnecessary travel. Reliability can exist even when a service is unavailable if information is honest and the alternative is clear. Brazil and Bolivia show that the community can be a partner, but the state remains responsible. Volunteers and local leaders are not substitutes for workforce and budget. Their role is to identify needs, mediate, and scrutinize. When a community must finance or operate a basic service alone, the right becomes dependent on local wealth. National solidarity is tested by the ability to move resources to places where need is great and the voice is weak.

Primary care as a foundation rather than an inferior service: a universal system can fail if people go directly to hospitals because the local clinic is unreliable. Strengthening primary care requires a stable team, medicines, suitable hours, and referral capacity. It should not be presented as a service for the poor while those who can afford to bypass it do so. Professional quality and continuing relationships can make it the center of the system. Family and community teams know living conditions and can prevent hospitalization, but they need specialist support and information. Community health workers can reach villages, identify high-risk pregnancy, monitor chronic illness, and translate between service and culture. Their role should be defined and paid. Reliance on untrained volunteers creates unstable service. When they transfer sensitive information, privacy within a small community must be protected. Local connection is an advantage, but also a risk if rules are absent.

Decentralization, Data, and Management Capacity

A local authority needs data to plan, but complex collection can burden a weak service. A small number of useful indicators should be selected and returned to managers and the community. A central system can provide infrastructure and support. If every authority defines measures differently, disparities cannot be identified. A national core is therefore needed alongside additional local information. Successful decentralization is not abandonment of standards, but distribution of decisions according to capacity and proximity to the problem. When an authority cannot manage a budget or procurement, central government should assist rather than punish residents. Support can include a professional team, joint procurement, and temporary oversight. A recovery process should be transparent and include an exit target. Responsibility then remains public rather than being rolled down to a weak community.

Traditional Midwives and Safe Referral

They do not need to become hospital employees, but trust can be built and a direct communication channel provided. Clinical teams should recognize their status in the community and avoid humiliation. At the same time, dangerous practices should be identified and an accessible alternative created. If referral leads to degrading treatment, cooperation will collapse. Safety also depends on how the woman is received in the institution. Consent during childbirth requires particular attention. Pain and urgency do not eliminate the need for explanation. When an interpreter or traditional companion is present, the woman herself remains the decision-maker as far as possible. A birth plan is not a contract that prevents change, but it helps the team understand preferences. After an emergency, the team should return and explain what was done.

Law and Budget in Accessible Language

A constitutional right can be used by organizations and communities to demand data and resources. To make the tool accessible, decisions should be published in language that is not purely legal. A map of services, travel time, and stock may be more powerful than a general statement. A court can require process or explanation, but implementation still needs follow-up by the public and authorities. A judgment that is not translated into budget and management may remain a symbolic achievement. Allocation should recognize that equality does not always mean equal distribution. A remote area may require higher cost to reach the same capacity. Compensatory financing is not favoritism; it corrects distance and history. The measure should be the result - access, health, and safety - rather than the same amount per resident. Transparent public discussion can explain why one area receives more without presenting that choice as discrimination.

A District Budget That Includes the Community

In a remote district, authorities must choose among expanding a permanent clinic, operating a mobile clinic, and providing transportation to a regional hospital. Rather than deciding only in the center, the authority publishes morbidity data, travel times, and costs, and discusses them with communities, professionals, and representatives of women and children.

Participation is not a popularity contest. Professionals define safety limits, while the community helps determine which barriers matter most and how the service should operate. After a year, travel times, referral completion, and service uptake are measured, and the budget is adjusted to the results.

The case shows how a social right is translated into transparent public choice. It does not guarantee every service in every place, but it requires reasons, participation, and reassessment.

Community Health Workers as a Bridge to the System

In remote areas, a community health worker can identify risk, follow treatment, and translate between the institution and daily life. The advantage is not that the worker is a cheap substitute for a physician, but familiarity with routes, language, and family. When the role is well defined, it reduces loss to follow-up and enables earlier referral to the appropriate place.

The risk is broad responsibility without training, pay, or support. A community worker should not face an emergency alone or carry blame for system shortages. A referral protocol, connection to a professional team, transportation, and documentation that continues with the patient are required.

Israel can apply the principle in remote or marginalized populations: a locally rooted figure with training and clearly defined authority, connected to the system rather than operating outside it.

Data Sovereignty of Indigenous Communities

Collecting health data about a community can improve planning but can also reproduce exploitation when information leaves the community, is used for research, or presents the community in a stigmatizing way. Data sovereignty seeks to give the community a voice in what is collected, who interprets it, how it is published, and what returns to the community.

This does not mean that individual rights are lost to the group. Individual consent is needed alongside community governance, especially when genetic or geographic data can identify relatives. Agreements should define ownership, access, retention period, and expected benefit.

Sharing results in a local language and useful format is part of fairness. An academic report that never reaches the community does not return the value taken from it. The principle applies to any population about which data are collected without an ability to influence their use.

Water, Sanitation, and Environment as the Boundary of Medicine

In Brazil and Bolivia, the right to health does not always begin in a clinic. Contaminated water, distance from a safe source, mining, smoke, and crowded housing can produce disease that clinical treatment repeatedly returns to the same environment. A system that finances medicine but fails to connect information with environmental health protects the individual only partially.

Indigenous and rural communities may detect changes in water, land, or illness patterns early, yet their information does not always enter official systems. A participation mechanism should allow community reporting, independent testing, and return of results in understandable language. Collecting samples without explanation, or using local knowledge without sharing results, repeats a pattern of extracting a resource from the community.

The division of responsibility among local authorities, health ministries, environmental agencies, and infrastructure bodies is itself a rights issue. When each body refers the family to another, the family is left with illness and no accountable address. A coordinating authority, timetable, and publication of corrective actions are needed. Remedies may include temporary water supply, monitoring, medical care, and compensation, not only a long-term report.

The lesson relevant to Israel is that health equity requires connecting the clinic, the local authority, and the environment. Regional morbidity data should trigger examination of living conditions rather than label the community a 'non-adherent population.'

Rights Navigation and Community Legal Assistance

A constitutional right or public insurance does not help a person who does not know why a request was denied, which document is missing, or where to appeal. In remote, Indigenous, or poor communities, the distance from law and administration may be as great as the distance from the clinic. Community navigation translates institutional language, helps collect documents, and identifies whether the problem is a local error or a broader pattern.

The navigator need not be a lawyer in every case. A trained community worker can solve registration, appointment, or referral problems; a lawyer is needed when there is a principled dispute, discrimination, or a need for an order. A graduated pathway reduces proceedings and prevents the court from becoming the only door to a basic medicine. At the same time, independence from the body whose decisions are being challenged should be preserved.

Accumulated information from inquiries can be used for oversight. If hundreds of people are required to submit the same document again, the problem is not patient incompetence but a defective process. Publishing anonymized patterns allows authorities to correct procedures before the dispute becomes a wave of litigation. The community should receive an answer about what changed, rather than having its stories used only as a data source.

The Israeli lesson is to build continuity among complaint commissioners, legal assistance, local authorities, and patient organizations. A community address can solve an early barrier, refer a complex case, and ensure that the person does not disappear between institutions. Access to a right then becomes a service in itself rather than a test of navigation skills.

Two Pathways for Realizing a Social Right in Latin America

Axis	**Brazil**	**Bolivia**	**Possible Lesson for Israel**
Anchoring the right	Constitution and SUS system	Broad right in a plurinational state	Connect a right with a clearly accountable implementing institution
Public participation	Health councils and	Representation of	Representation with

Axis	Brazil	Bolivia	Possible Lesson for Israel
	local mechanisms	communities and different identities	information and authority, not ritual
Access in the periphery	Primary care and decentralization	Distance, infrastructure, and integration of traditions	Measure travel time and continuity of service
Law and budget	Claims for medicines and services	More limited enforcement capacity	Assess the group impact of individual relief
Culture and care	Accommodation within a public system	Explicit intercultural health	Combine cultural choice with safety rules

The distinctive feature of the Latin American comparison is the question of who participates in realizing the right. Brazil and Bolivia emphasize community, territory, and living conditions. The lesson for Israel is to ask whether there is a local accountable address, whether regional data change decisions, and whether participation has influence before a dispute reaches court. The comparison therefore tests not only the right itself, but also a community's ability to influence priorities.

Chapter Eleven: North America - United States and Canada

Opening Dilemma

An American patient and a Canadian patient both need advanced imaging. The American receives a quick appointment but discovers that the provider is out of network and the cost is high; the Canadian is covered but must wait. Both are constrained, but in different ways. An operational right requires the American system to provide reliable network and cost information before the decision, and the Canadian system to provide information about time, priority, and alternatives. The comparison shows that it is not enough to say there is choice or there is coverage. The question is what a person can actually do at the moment the service is needed. The scenario highlights that autonomy and access are separate axes. A system can protect consent well while leaving people without care, or guarantee coverage without providing conversation and explanation.

The same right to refuse does not confer the same ability to receive.

The United States and Canada share a legal tradition of autonomy but differ profoundly in financing: a fragmented market and insurance structure versus provincial public insurance under federal principles.

1. United States: Strong Autonomy and a Fragmented System

American law played a central role in developing informed consent, privacy, and the right to refuse, but the ability to receive routine care depends heavily on insurance, employment, income, and state of residence. Judicial doctrines concerning bodily integrity and informed consent predated

Medicare and Medicaid. Later reforms expanded coverage but did not create a single universal system.

At the organizational level, hospitals, insurers, employers, states, and the federal government divide responsibility. Fragmentation can permit innovation and choice for part of the population, but it also creates complexity and administrative costs. A patient may receive an excellent explanation of alternatives and still choose according to copayments and provider networks. Medical choice occurs within an economic framework.

A market can increase availability of technology but also encourage overtreatment. Consumer rights do not correct a disparity when a person cannot purchase the service. Israel adopted some of the American language of autonomy while preserving universal insurance. Maintaining that distinction is important as private financing expands.

The lesson for Israel is to protect consent and rights-based law without allowing the market to make access to care dependent on purchasing power.

2. EMTALA and the Minimum Right in an Emergency

Key sources: 42 U.S.C. § 1395dd; CMS, 2026.

EMTALA prohibits covered hospitals from refusing emergency screening and stabilizing treatment because of ability to pay, but it is not comprehensive health insurance. Historically, the 1986 federal law was enacted in response to patient dumping - transferring or refusing uninsured patients. It requires a medical screening examination and stabilization or an appropriate transfer.

Institutionally, the duty applies to emergency departments of hospitals participating in Medicare, which includes most hospitals. It protects anyone who presents, not only Medicare beneficiaries. An uninsured person will receive stabilizing treatment for a myocardial infarction but may afterward face a high bill and difficulty obtaining follow-up. The right prevents immediate abandonment but does not ensure continuity.

The gap between principle and implementation nonetheless remains. The law functions as a safety net but burdens emergency departments when community access is inadequate. An emergency duty is not a substitute for accessible primary care. In Israel, the Patients' Rights Law establishes a duty to provide urgent treatment without prior conditions within a universal insurance system. The comparison highlights the importance of connecting the emergency gateway with continuing coverage.

An emergency right should include coordination of follow-up and financial protection. Otherwise it saves the moment while leaving the illness and the debt behind.

3. Canada: The Canada Health Act and the Principles of Medicare

Key source: Canada Health Act, R.S.C. 1985, c. C-6.

The Canada Health Act links federal funding to the principles of public administration, comprehensiveness, universality, portability, and accessibility, and protects against charges for insured services. Historically, the system developed at the provincial level, and the 1984 federal law consolidated principles as conditions for fiscal transfers. Responsibility for delivery and management remained largely provincial.

In practice, insured services mainly include medically necessary physician and hospital care. Community drugs, dental care, and other services are covered variably. A patient may pay nothing at the point of service for an insured operation, yet wait a long time or pay for medication outside the hospital. Universality is not absolute comprehensiveness.

Restrictions on extra billing protect equality, but waiting times fuel debate about private provision. The question is whether private supply adds capacity or draws personnel from the public system. In Israel, Canadian principles are close to the values of the National Health Insurance Law. Supplementary and private insurance play a broader role in Israel and therefore require scrutiny of their impact on equality.

The public package should be defined clearly, waiting times published, and hidden charges prevented. Equality at the point of service also depends on reasonable availability.

4. Autonomy Within Similar Legal Cultures

In both countries, rights to consent, confidentiality, and refusal became established, but economic organization shapes the ability to use those rights and the points of conflict. Canadian case law and provincial charters, alongside American law, strengthened end-of-life decision-making, information rights, and accountability. The medical profession moved toward partnership in a manner similar to Israel.

In the clinical arena, the central barrier in the United States may be insurance coverage; in Canada it may be availability and waiting. In both cases, the patient encounters a limit that is not set only by the physician. A right to a second opinion is not equivalent when the specialist is out of network or when the next appointment is months away. The right needs infrastructure.

No system eliminates rationing completely. The question is whether rationing is by price, time, medical criteria, or a combination, and how transparent it is. Israel combines public waiting, supplementary insurance, and private medicine and therefore carries features of both systems. This creates a risk of double rationing by both time and money.

Coverage alone should not be measured; time, out-of-pocket spending, and ability to use an alternative should also be measured. Clinical rights must be examined inside the real economy.

5. Lessons for Israel: Universality, Market Boundaries, and Transparency

The comparison shows that a system can be advanced in autonomy but weak in access, or universal but limited in availability. Israel should protect both dimensions. Historically, North American reforms show how difficult fragmentation is to correct once it becomes entrenched, and how public rights require continued protection against charges and bypass routes.

For institutions, public financing should come with accountability for results; private financing should be regulated so that it does not damage the public workforce or queue. A private route that shortens the wait to the same specialist, for example, may expand choice for one person while lengthening the wait for others. Policy must measure the system-wide effect.

A complete ban on private care may be unrealistic, but unlimited acceptance can create two systems. Rules are needed on dual practice, queues, and information. Israel's advantage is universal coverage and longitudinal health-fund records; its weakness is rising private expenditure and disparities. The advantage should not be lost in an effort to shorten waits.

A policy goal should be access according to need, within a reasonable time and with financial protection, alongside autonomy. Every reform should be measured against all three criteria together.

Financing and Choice: Insurance Coverage and Financial Risk

Medical choice does not occur in a vacuum. Provider networks, prior authorization, medical debt, distance, and waiting can change the practical alternative even when the clinical decision is clear. This section compares financing constraints in the

United States and Canada and translates them into questions relevant to Israel.

Medical Choice Within an Insurance Contract

Before a major decision, the insurance implications should also be explained when known, or the patient should be referred to someone who can clarify them. Physicians should not be expected to know every policy, but institutions should recognize that price is part of the decision rather than an external administrative matter. American informed-consent law contributed to a move from what the customary physician would disclose toward information material to the patient. This strengthened choice but sometimes produced long forms and defensive medicine. When the discussion centers on a list of risks for legal protection, the person may receive more details while understanding less. Good implementation connects disclosure to preferences: which risk changes the decision, what are the alternatives, and what happens without treatment. The law then serves the conversation rather than replacing it. Federal privacy rules created protections for use of medical information, but their boundaries do not cover every app, digital service, or company holding health data. A person may provide data to a smartwatch without understanding that those data are not protected in the same way as a medical record. The split between medical law and consumer law creates a gray area. A health system should explain when it refers a patient to an external tool, limit collection, and review terms of use. General consent to an app is not a substitute for responsibility by the institution that recommended it.

The cost of a fragmented market: the harm is not only to health; it changes bargaining power in the room. A person who fears a bill does not ask the same questions or choose freely. An unexpected charge can turn successful treatment into a financial crisis. Price transparency is necessary, but a system in which the price depends on network status, coding, and a complex contract is not solved by a list on a website. Human assistance, advance planning, and limits on surprises are needed where there was no real opportunity to choose. Litigation can compensate and expose failure, but it is expensive, slow, and inaccessible to many. Complaint mechanisms, disclosure of errors, and administrative compensation may provide an earlier response. They should be independent enough to examine the institution but connected closely enough to enable correction. The existence of a right to sue does not remove the duty to explain and learn. Rights protection is not measured by the number of lawyers but by a person's ability to obtain an answer and correction without spending years in proceedings.

Canada: Universality with Limits

Waiting for consultations and procedures also creates a gap between entitlement and availability. Patients need information about the queue, urgency, and alternatives, not only reassurance that they are insured. The division of responsibility between federation and provinces permits adaptation but creates variation. A person moving between regions may encounter different rules and services. Formal portability should be accompanied by information transfer and continuity. When treatment is delayed, there should be a way to review priority rather than simply wait. A fair waiting list requires clinical criteria, updates, and transparency about changes. Indigenous health in Canada exposes the limits of universality. Public coverage can coexist with distance, discrimination, and memory of harmful institutions. Access requires local service, cultural safety, and community participation. Distrust is not resolved by saying the service is equal for everyone. One must examine how it is delivered, who makes decisions, and whether patients can criticize care without fear. History changes the meaning of the encounter even when the current procedure appears neutral.

The same diagnosis, two constraints: good policy should connect them. When a clinical option depends on cost or waiting, that limitation should enter the conversation. This is not turning the physician into an insurance agent; it is recognizing that a decision that cannot be carried out is not a complete choice.

What can be measured and transferred to Israel: comparison requires more than insurance rates. It should examine foregone care because of cost, waiting times, medical debt, access to complaint mechanisms, continuity, and understanding of options. Breakdown by income, geography, and ethnic group reveals whether rights can be used equally. Complaint volume by itself is not a performance measure; more informative measures include the type of harm, response time, proportion of cases leading to correction, and whether different groups use the route similarly. Numbers therefore need to be read alongside experiences and explanations of reporting rules. The lesson for Israel is to preserve public universality while examining how a private market changes queues, workforce, and decisions. When a patient is referred to a private route, the public alternative and expected time should be explained. Choice then does not exploit the person's uncertainty. Israel could also strengthen complaint and compensation mechanisms that do not depend on lengthy litigation, especially around clear errors, billing, or delay. Such mechanisms should publish principles, response times, and what changed following complaints. At the same time, staff should be protected from defensive medicine through a culture of disclosure and learning. A system that hides errors increases litigation; a system that acknowledges and corrects them can preserve trust.

Choosing Among Providers and Information That Is Not Comparable

A list of providers is not necessarily choice. Patients need to know who is available, service quality, expected cost, and travel distance. In the American system such information is scattered among insurers, hospitals, and public databases; in Canada, choice may be more limited, but there are still differences among institutions and regions. Independent navigation can turn data into a decision. A sick person should not be expected to analyze contracts and quality indicators alone. Quality itself is not a single number. Complication rates, experience, patient-reported experience, and continuity may point in different directions. Publication should present several measures and explain their limitations. Overly simple rankings encourage institutions to select easier patients or improve the measure rather than the care. A conversation with a professional can help determine what matters to the individual. Choice is a process of matching, not an ordinary consumer competition.

Emergency Care and a Charge That Could Not Be Chosen: in an emergency, a person cannot check network status or price. A high bill after immediately necessary care undermines the idea of contractual consent. Protection against surprise billing seeks to separate financial disputes between provider and insurer from the patient. Even where law restricts charging, institutions should explain rights and assist with appeals. An automatically generated threatening letter can cause harm before the dispute is resolved. In Canada, direct payment is smaller in emergencies, but interprovincial care or an uninsured service may still create uncertainty. Portability requires coordination, not only a principle. A person traveling or moving should know how coverage works and what documents to retain. When one body pays and another treats, the administrative dispute should not delay care. Inter-institutional responsibility protects the person from fragmentation.

Indigenous Health and Sovereignty over Information

Indigenous communities in North America have demanded not only access to services but control over how their data are collected and used. Research or information systems can generate conclusions about a community without returning benefits or allowing local interpretation. Principles of ownership, control, access, and possession seek to correct this. The point is not to abolish research but to create partnership that defines purpose, authorization, and publication. Culturally safe care is also measured by the experience of treatment. A one-time training session about customs is insufficient if a person encounters racism or assumptions. Organizations should allow reporting, examine care disparities, and include professionals from the community. Telemedicine can bring specialist expertise, but reliable local service remains essential. Trust is built over time through presence, accountability, and recognition of history.

What Can Be Learned About Supplementary and Private Insurance in Israel

The North American comparison warns against a system in which the private layer effectively determines speed of access. In Israel, public insurance remains the foundation, but multiple pathways can create confusion and pressure to purchase. Public information should clarify what is included in the statutory basket, what is available through supplementary insurance, and what is private. When the same physician works in multiple settings, safeguards are needed against referrals that exploit an information gap. Monitoring should examine not only how many people are insured but whether private use changes public availability. Data on working hours, queues, and workforce movement can reveal effects. One should not assume that every private activity is harmful, but neither should it be assumed to be separate. Rights policy must view the system as a whole and ensure that one person's choice does not make another person's wait unreasonable.

Prior Authorization and a Decision That Does Not Begin in the Physician's Room

In the American system, a clinical decision may pass through an additional insurer review. Prior authorization is intended to reduce unnecessary care, but when criteria are not transparent it shifts power from the professional treating the body to an organization that never meets the person. A patient who hears from the physician that treatment is recommended and then receives an administrative denial may not understand who made the decision or on what basis. A practical right requires a reasoned notice, an expedited appeal route in urgent cases, and institutional responsibility to help transfer documents. It is not enough to say that the insurer refused; the patient should be told what is missing, who can provide it, and what clinical alternative exists in the meantime. Staff also pay a cost when hours are spent on calls and forms. This burden is not merely an efficiency problem: it reduces time for conversation, delays care, and rewards those who know how to navigate the system. Proper measurement should examine time to decision, reversal rates on appeal, effect on treatment initiation, and disparities among groups. If most denials are overturned, the quality of the initial decision should be examined rather than merely celebrating successful appeals. A good mechanism reduces the need for struggle instead of making struggle a condition of receiving care.

Medical Debt as a Failure of Autonomy

Medical debt is not merely a secondary economic consequence. It can affect housing, credit, employment, and willingness to seek future care. A person asked to choose treatment without knowing its real cost does not have full consent in the social sense of the term, even if the medical explanation was excellent. Transparency should be provided before planned care but cannot become a condition for life-saving treatment. After emergency care, an assistance pathway is needed that is not humiliating and does not assume that every person can negotiate. Hospitals can publish discount policies, offer counseling, and review whether an unusual charge matches the information given. In Canada, the financial barrier is smaller for insured services but does not disappear in areas outside the provincial basket. A person may receive surgery without charge and struggle to finance medicines, rehabilitation, or dental care that affects health. The gap between hospital and community is, in a sense, similar to the gap between coverage and availability.

The full journey should therefore be examined rather than asking only whether the visit itself was public. Rights policy should identify costs that prevent continuation of care and offer information and referral before discharge.

Telemedicine and North American Distance

In rural and remote areas, telemedicine can reduce travel and bring specialist expertise. It is not an automatic substitute for physical examination, privacy, or a continuing relationship. The system should ask whether the patient has a connection, a device, and a quiet space and can use them. Technical failure should not be treated as failure to attend. In Indigenous communities, remote services should be integrated with a local team and clear rules on ownership and use of data. Otherwise technology reproduces distance instead of bridging it. Choice between remote and in-person care should be based on clinical need and patient preference, not only provider convenience. When a remote visit is insufficient, a rapid transition to a physical pathway should be guaranteed rather than requiring the patient to start over. Measures such as resolution of the problem, conversion to an additional visit, satisfaction, and digital disparities provide a better picture than call volume alone. This permits use of the tool without turning it into a gate that excludes the very people who need care.

Clinically Approved Treatment but Insurance Denied

A physician recommends a medicine, but the insurer requires a prior trial of another drug. She explains the reason for the denial and the risk of delay, files an expedited appeal with documentation, and arranges a temporary alternative. The patient receives updates and is not required to manage the conversation alone. In a Canadian system, a parallel scenario may be a long wait for consultation. There too, someone should update the patient, assess deterioration, and offer transfer where possible. The systems differ, but in both the right is tested by how the gap between need and availability is managed. The comparison also clarifies the role of economic information. Institutions should identify in advance where costs are likely and refer patients for assistance. Clinicians do not need to calculate bills, but should know that cost can alter a plan. The North American lesson is that even in wealthy systems the barrier can move from the door to the contract, from price to waiting, and from distance to technology. Rights policy should follow the entire pathway rather than stop at coverage rates. A person needs actionable information, an accountable address when the promise fails, and protection from a price that could not reasonably have been anticipated. Freedom of choice without ability to pay may be empty, and coverage without availability may be frustrating and dangerous. A practical right is created by connecting information, financing, time, and correction.

An American patient receives a recommendation for two medicines with similar effectiveness, but only after the visit discovers that one is outside the insurance formulary and will cost hundreds of dollars per month. Clinically, alternatives were presented; practically, there was no real choice. A conversation that includes expected cost, authorization requirements, and the appeal route in advance can prevent treatment abandonment. In Canada, the constraint may be different - a prolonged wait for a specialist. In both situations, the access limitation should be disclosed as information relevant to the decision rather than as a later administrative surprise.

Expected Price as Part of Informed Consent: In a system where treatment may generate debt, medical information alone is not sufficient for choice. Patients need to know not only the clinical risk of a procedure but also what is likely to be covered, the expected cost-sharing, and which providers may bill separately. An estimate is not always exact, but total absence of information makes consent incomplete.

Price transparency is not a list of thousands of tariffs that no one can interpret. What is needed is a personalized estimate, distinction between planned and emergency care, and an address for clarification. Where coverage is uncertain, the institution can flag financial risk before treatment and offer an appropriate clinical alternative, payment plan, or eligibility assistance. A cheaper alternative should not be presented as medically superior when it is not.

Canada and other public systems also contain costs that are not always covered - medicines outside hospital, transportation, dental care, or lost work. Protection against financial harm therefore requires looking at the whole pathway rather than only the price of the visit. A patient who abandons follow-up because of indirect cost has not realized in practice the right received in the hospital.

Israel has room to expand information about the costs of private services, supplementary insurance, medicines, and travel. The purpose is not to turn the physician into a financial adviser, but to ensure that someone in the system explains a material price before the person becomes locked into a decision.

Employment-Based Insurance and Continuity During Job Change

In the United States, the link between insurance and employment creates a dependence unrelated to clinical need. A person may remain in a job to preserve treatment, postpone a move, or fear dismissal during illness. Clinical choice is therefore influenced by whether coverage will continue, which physicians will remain in network, and what the transition will cost.

Job loss may occur precisely when need for treatment increases. Clear notice of when coverage ends, continuation options, and transfer of authorizations can prevent interruption of medicines and tests. A general brochure is not enough; a patient in active treatment needs a plan identifying what must be completed, what can be transferred, and who is responsible for the documents.

Continuity also depends on portability of information. When a new physician cannot quickly obtain a summary, results, and medication authorization, changing insurance becomes a restart. A system that allows patients to download a usable record and transfer it reduces dependence on the contract between insurer and provider.

The comparison highlights for Israel that changes between employers, health funds, supplementary insurance, or eligibility frameworks can also disrupt continuity. The right does not require every arrangement to remain identical, but it does require notice, a transition period, and a practical way to prevent dangerous interruption.

How Financing Shapes Patients' Rights in North America

Dimension	**United States**	**Canada**	**Implication for Israel**
Financial barrier	Cost-sharing and debt	Broad public coverage for insured services	Examine total cost, not only formal entitlement
Choice of provider	Limited by network and insurance authorization	Less extensive choice in some areas and dependent on waiting	Present time, distance, and cost in the same interface
Emergency care	Stabilization duty alongside possible billing	Public access without payment at the point of care	Separate immediate treatment from later billing disputes
Telemedicine	Diverse, market-based, and non-uniform solutions	A tool for reducing distance in a public system	Ensure continuity and privacy across channels
Indigenous populations	Trust and access disparities	Questions of sovereignty and adapted service	Combine control over data with community partnership

The North American comparison sharpens the point that autonomy also depends on coverage, price, and availability. In the United States, financial risk is more prominent; in Canada, waiting may be the more central limitation. In Israel, choice should also be examined by asking what can actually be realized, what it will cost, and how long a person will have to wait.

Chapter Twelve: Asia - China, Japan, Thailand, and Malaysia

Opening Dilemma

An older patient with advanced illness arrives at a hospital while her son asks the team not to speak with her about the end of life. He explains that in their family difficult decisions are made together and that a direct conversation would damage hope. Also in the room are a nurse who knows the patient and a spiritual-care representative. The first step is not to choose between 'culture' and 'rights,' but to ask the patient how she wants to receive information, who should participate, and what is important for her to preserve. She may ask that her son hear the details and help her decide; she may prefer a private conversation; or she may choose gradual disclosure. A request to involve family or faith can itself be an expression of autonomy, provided that it comes from the patient and can be changed. When the preference is unknown, professional responsibility is to create a space in which it can be explored without pressure and without stereotype.

Tradition can offer a language for decision-making; it must not make the decision in place of the person.

The four countries in this chapter present different ways of connecting health coverage, professional authority, family, religion, and rights mechanisms. China and Japan illuminate the effects of institutions, ageing, and coordination; Thailand adds universal coverage, rights protection, and a Buddhist discourse on suffering and the end of life; Malaysia adds a public-private system and a multireligious Muslim-majority society. The comparison does not seek a single 'Asian model,' but examines how common principles take different forms.

1. Four Asias - Not One Culture

The term 'Asia' includes countries with very different histories, regimes, religions, economies, and health systems. Using a single label may turn family orientation, obedience, or spirituality into a fixed trait attributed to a person solely because of origin. The comparison is useful precisely when it separates three layers: system structure, social norms, and individual preference. Each layer influences the encounter, but none alone predicts what a patient will want.

Family plays a central role in all four countries, but for different reasons. Sometimes it is the main source of support in an overloaded system; sometimes it expresses a conception of intergenerational responsibility; and sometimes it is needed to bridge language, transportation, or cost. Such involvement can expand the ability to choose, but it can also create pressure, concealment of information, or transfer of the burden of care from the state to the home.

Religion is not a clinical category either. Buddhism in Thailand and Islam in Malaysia provide concepts of compassion, suffering, duty, hope, and death, but there are different streams and interpretations, and many people combine faith with secular or medical positions. A staff member does not need to be an expert in every tradition; the staff member needs to know how to ask, listen, and invite spiritual consultation when the patient wants it.

The comparative framework therefore rests on recurring questions: who finances and organizes the service, how the patient obtains information and redress, who participates in the decision, how privacy is protected, and what happens when a family or religious value conflicts with a medical recommendation. The questions are the same; the institutional answers differ.

2. China: Scale, Trust, and Data Governance

China has expanded coverage and services on an enormous scale, but use of the system is often concentrated in large hospitals. When community medicine is not perceived as a sufficient point of care, patients go directly to crowded centers, and the brief encounter becomes the place where expectations for diagnosis, treatment, and explanation accumulate. Such overload is not merely an inconvenience; it reduces time for conversation and increases the risk that a decision will be perceived as arbitrary.

Trust is also affected by incentives. A patient who suspects that a recommendation is linked to income, testing, or personal connections finds it difficult to view the physician as neutral. Transparency in payment, separation between consultation and sale, and stronger primary care matter to rights no less than a consent form. When the explanation is given within a system perceived as unfair, a signature does not repair the crisis of trust.

Extensive digitization creates advantages in continuity, scheduling, and access to information, but it also concentrates large volumes of data in institutions and platforms. The rights question moves from who knows the diagnosis to who may use the data, for what purpose, and how an automated decision can be challenged. A family member who manages an older person's account may help, but authorization should be graduated rather than allowing convenience to become unlimited control.

The lesson is not that state authority or technology necessarily harms rights. A large system can set standards, make information accessible, and identify gaps rapidly. The condition is that complaint, review, and explanation mechanisms operate alongside efficiency, and that performance data do not replace a person's ability to ask why a decision was made about them.

3. Japan: Universality, Choice, and Ageing

Japan has operated universal health insurance since 1961 through multiple plans and a nationally regulated fee schedule. Broad provider choice facilitates access, but it can also produce repeated visits and fragmentation among specialists. A person with chronic illnesses can receive correct decisions in every clinic and still accumulate medicines, tests, and recommendations that do not form a single plan.

Population ageing shifts the focus of rights from an acute event to a long continuum: support at home, rehabilitation, nursing care, place of residence, and end-of-life planning. Capacity may change gradually, so a one-time decision about who represents the person is insufficient. Values need to be documented, ability assessed in relation to each decision, and the person included even when support is needed.

A tradition of respect for authority and harmony can support trust, but can also reduce questioning. Professional change does not require encouraging confrontation; it requires a clear invitation to ask questions and disagree. A physician who presents a recommendation and explains that another choice is permitted preserves professional authority while also opening a space for autonomy.

Family members often carry a substantial burden of care. A plan that assumes unlimited availability of children or spouses presents a choice that may not be realizable. Rights in old age include assessment of family capacity, respite services, professional coordination, and recognition that preventing overtreatment can protect quality of life rather than represent withdrawal from care.

4. Thailand: Universal Coverage, Rights Protection, and the End of Life

Key sources: Thailand National Health Act, 2007; WHO, 2019.

Thailand achieved universal health coverage through three public schemes, including the Universal Coverage Scheme for people not covered by the others. The achievement is not merely an expansion of insurance; it built an administrative mechanism that defines the benefits package, provider payment, and rights protection. Complaint channels and rights centers allow people to clarify entitlement, complain, and obtain assistance without beginning with litigation.

An accessible rights mechanism changes power relations. A patient who does not receive a service need not know which court has jurisdiction; the patient can approach an administrative address that knows the system. To be credible, the mechanism must be able to follow correction, publish patterns, and distinguish a dispute about the benefits package from a failure of implementation. A hotline that collects complaints but cannot influence providers creates another layer of disappointment.

Thai law also recognizes the possibility of writing a directive refusing a service whose sole purpose is to prolong the dying process or prolong suffering in a terminal condition. In recent years digital tools have been added to make such directives more accessible. The ethical meaning extends beyond the document: end of life becomes a subject for an earlier conversation about goals, palliative care, and who will interpret the person's wishes if the person cannot speak.

Buddhist concepts of impermanence, compassion, and reduction of suffering may help some patients and families, but they should not automatically be taken to imply a preference to forgo treatment. A religious person may request aggressive treatment, and a nonreligious person may request avoidance of burdensome intervention. A monk or spiritual companion participates only with the patient's consent and does not replace medical assessment or consent.

Thailand shows that coverage, an administrative right, and end-of-life planning can exist within the same framework.

Challenges remain in regional disparities, workload, access for migrants, and groups whose status is unclear. A universal right is tested most sharply for those who do not know how to present a document, speak the language, or navigate among schemes.

5. Malaysia: A Hybrid System and a Multireligious Muslim-Majority Society

Key sources: Ministry of Health Malaysia, 2023; MMC, 2025.

Malaysia operates a hybrid system: a broad public service, financed mainly from state revenues and providing highly subsidized care, alongside a substantial private sector. The division creates options but also queues, workforce movement, and differences in availability. The right is tested not only by whether a public hospital exists, but whether care can be obtained there within a reasonable time without the private pathway becoming the default for those who can pay.

Most of Malaysia's population is Muslim, alongside Buddhist, Christian, Hindu, and other communities. This religious diversity prevents an assumption that the system can operate according to a single cultural code. The treatment room may include different preferences regarding the sex of the caregiver, food, prayer, privacy, touch, disclosure of information, and the end of life. A uniform standard should guarantee respect, while adaptation is made to the individual.

Guidance of the Malaysian Medical Council emphasizes autonomy, informed consent, and confidentiality as professional duties. This creates a layer of protection that does not depend only on a separate patients' rights statute. Its advantage is professional flexibility; its disadvantage is that the patient may find it difficult to know what remedy exists when the guidance is breached. Clear complaint mechanisms, public information, and a distinction between disciplinary proceedings and immediate resolution of a clinical need are therefore required.

Malaysia's Ministry of Health promotes advance care planning and conversations with patients and their loved ones about treatments they would want or refuse if their condition worsens. The framework emphasizes conversation, documentation, and the possibility of change, but its legal status is not identical in every respect to that of a binding statutory directive. Consistent documentation, designation of a trusted person, and agreement across teams are therefore especially important.

Islamic ethics can distinguish between the duty to preserve life and treatment that is futile or excessively burdensome, and can give weight to intention, suffering, and family duty. There is no automatic religious answer to every case. When the patient requests it, a religious adviser familiar with medicine may be involved; the decision remains a clinical-ethical process that respects the patient's wishes, the law, and professional boundaries.

6. Comparative View: Four Systems, Five Tests

The comparison reveals five separate tests. The first is access: does coverage enable treatment to be obtained, or does it merely provide formal entitlement? The second is coordination: can a person move among physician, hospital, home care, and nursing care without becoming the sole manager of the case? The third is redress: is there a simple address capable of correcting a problem rather than merely recording a complaint?

The fourth test is decision-making style. China and Japan, in different ways, emphasize relationships and family; Thailand and Malaysia add a more visible religious and spiritual language in some cases. In all four countries, the proper decision begins by clarifying the person's preference rather than assuming it on the basis of nationality, age, or religion.

The fifth test is the boundary of family responsibility. Family can translate, support, provide care, and preserve continuity, but it is not a substitute for financing, workforce, or the patient's decision. When the state transfers care to the home, it should offer training, equipment, respite, and an available point of contact. Otherwise, the language of tradition conceals an institutional cutback.

Israel has similarities to each of these countries: a broad public system, choice among providers, involved families, religious groups, and a multilingual society. The lesson is not to adopt one national model, but to build a process that clarifies preference, documents it, enables redress, and verifies that the choice is feasible in terms of resources.

Cross-Cultural Implementation: Family, Faith, and the End of Life

A high-quality cross-cultural encounter is not a list of customs. It is a process that identifies who the person is, which relationships and beliefs matter, and the point at which support becomes pressure. At the end of life, this process should begin early, before crisis reduces time and capacity.

Religion is a question, not a ready-made answer: an open question such as, 'Is there a belief, practice, or spiritual person that is important for us to take into account?' allows patients to define what religion means for them. There is no need to begin with the name of a denomination or assume a position about the soul, pain, or treatment. A person can choose one practice and reject another, and the preference may change as illness progresses.

Spiritual information is documented only to the extent necessary for care and with consent. A label such as 'Muslim' or 'Buddhist' is not a clinical instruction. Documentation should be concrete: requests time for prayer, prefers a particular adviser, does not want prognosis discussed without a daughter present, or asks that a medical decision first be explained to the patient alone.

Family as a source of knowledge and a source of pressure: a family member knows habits, values, and subtle changes, and is sometimes the only person able to provide support at home. The team should therefore listen even when the family member lacks formal authority. At the same time, the team should create a moment in which the patient can speak without family present, if the patient wishes. A brief private space may reveal a preference that has been swallowed by concern or hierarchy.

When family members disagree, a representative should not be selected according to age, sex, or the loudest voice. The team examines what the patient said previously, who was designated, who cared for the patient, and whether there are conflicts of interest. Mediation is intended to return the disagreement to values and medical information, not to decide which family member is more worthy.

Thailand: An Advance Directive as Part of a Conversation About Suffering

A written directive can reduce treatment that prolongs the dying process contrary to a person's wishes, but its value depends on the conversation that preceded it. The team should clarify what the person understands as a terminal condition, which abilities are essential to that person, and what the person would regard as intolerable suffering. A list of procedures alone cannot cover an unforeseen scenario.

When a directive is activated, palliative care, presence, food, hygiene, and support for the family do not stop. A clear distinction between avoiding burdensome intervention and abandonment is essential to trust. The language of a 'good death' can help, but it should rest on the person's wishes rather than pressure to save resources.

Malaysia: Advance Care Planning Within Religious Diversity

Advance care planning in Malaysia is structured as a conversation among the person, loved ones, and the care team about future goals and preferences. In a multireligious society, the document should avoid language that assumes one conception of duty or death. It can include who should advise spiritually, who should receive information, and what the team should do if the family requests treatment that the patient rejected.

When a care plan does not have the same legal status as a binding order in every situation, the importance of the process increases: updating the record, making it accessible across settings, repeating the conversation, and confirming a trusted decision-maker. The more the system is divided between public and private care, the more it needs a portable format that does not remain in one institution's file.

A spiritual adviser as a limited partner: an imam, monk, priest, or other adviser can translate concepts, reduce fear, and help a family understand that palliative care is not abandonment. Participation requires the patient's consent, protection of confidentiality, and clarification that the adviser is not authorized to change a medical decision or speak for the person without authorization.

The institution should maintain a pool of advisers familiar with privacy, consent, and end-of-life rules. Reliance on a person brought only by the family may be appropriate, but in a dispute a neutral person is also needed. Consultation is measured by its ability to expand understanding and reduce pressure, not by the number of visits.

Refusal of Treatment Is Not Refusal of Relationship

A patient who refuses ventilation, dialysis, or surgery is still entitled to explanation, pain treatment, nursing care, and follow-up. Withdrawal by the team or a statement that 'there is nothing more to do' punishes the patient for the choice and deepens the family's fear. The team should explain what will still be done, who will remain responsible, and when a decision can be changed.

Agreement to aggressive treatment is not the end of the discussion either. A review point, desired outcome, and condition for reassessing benefit should be set. This preserves hope without turning a temporary intervention into a pathway from which there is no exit.

Minorities, migrants, and people without status: national coverage can still leave outside effective access those who lack documents, struggle with language, or fear an authority. Thailand and Malaysia face migrant populations and groups with changing status; the gap is especially visible in primary care, pregnancy, communicable disease, and emergency care. Late presentation increases risk and cost for the entire system.

Multilingual explanation, separation between care and immigration enforcement where appropriate, a community point of contact, and documentation that does not disclose more than necessary are required. The right does not require every pathway to be identical, but it does require that a difference in status not become a preventable danger.

Comparative Case: A Request to Stop Ventilation

A competent patient with advanced illness asks that ventilation not be continued if the patient cannot return to basic communication. The family objects: some rely on a religious duty to preserve life, while others fear guilt. The team documents the patient's values, explains the prognosis, and proposes a defined trial point. Spiritual consultation is invited only after the patient agrees.

In Thailand, the conversation can be connected to an advance directive and the right to avoid a service that prolongs the dying process. In Malaysia, advance care planning, professional guidance, and clinical-ethical consultation can be used. The legal difference matters, but the order of work is similar: wishes, capacity, information, documentation, palliative care, and protection from pressure.

If the patient loses capacity before the disagreement is resolved, the decision rests on what the patient said, not on a family vote. A spiritual adviser can explain that stopping every treatment need not be equated with causing death; the medical team should explain what futile treatment means and what is expected after it is withdrawn. The conversation does not eliminate moral pain, but prevents that pain from erasing the person at the center.

What to measure in a cross-cultural encounter: a quality indicator cannot consist only of the number of referrals to a religious adviser. It should examine whether information preferences were asked about, whether participation in decision-making was documented, whether time for private conversation was provided, and whether the plan traveled across settings. Complaints about concealment of information or family pressure should be examined alongside complaints about lack of spiritual sensitivity.

A short survey can ask whether the person felt that the team respected beliefs without assuming them, and whether family members understood the limits of their role. Record review should examine accessibility of advance directives and care planning. When indicators are stratified by language, region, and status, it becomes possible to see whether cultural adaptation is available only to those who know how to demand it.

Lessons for Israel

Israel does not need to import religious or institutional language from another country. It can adopt three principles: ask before assuming, document decision-making style and not only the decision, and build a stable connection among clinical care, spiritual support, and a redress mechanism. These principles fit a Jewish, Muslim, Christian, Druze, and secular society without giving one group control over another.

An accessible administrative complaint mechanism, portable advance care planning, and family support are complementary components. They protect the patient, but also the team that today is often required to resolve, alone and during crisis, a medical, religious, and family dispute. The aim is not to remove difficulty, but to distribute responsibility and create a course of action that can be explained and reviewed.

Thailand: Early Assistance After Harm Without Waiting for Proof of Fault

Key source: Thailand National Health Security Act, 2002, s. 41.

Under Thailand's Universal Coverage Scheme, a mechanism provides initial financial assistance to people harmed by medical services. Its purpose is not to determine in advance whether negligence occurred, but to provide an early response to the harm and the resulting need. Distinguishing assistance from a judgment allows a family to receive support without waiting years for a complex proceeding.

Such a mechanism changes the language of response. Instead of viewing every approach as a legal threat, an institution can acknowledge harm and investigate it in parallel. Assistance does not remove the need for investigation, correction, or professional accountability; nor should it bar a claim where a cause of action exists. Its role is to reduce the cost of time and the need to prove fault as a condition for any help.

Fairness requires published criteria, a decision time, an appeal option, and an explanation of the relationship between assistance and other pathways. If the amount or procedure is unclear, the mechanism may be perceived as an attempt to buy silence. Publication of anonymized data on types of harm can also turn applications into a source of learning.

For Israel, the relevant question is whether, in some cases, immediate support can be separated from legal determination. A fund or limited institutional pathway could reduce distress and strengthen disclosure, provided that it does not replace investigation and transparency.

Malaysia: Professional Complaint, Institutional Complaint, and Civil Claim

In Malaysia, as in many countries, there is no single address for every kind of harm. A complaint against a physician may go to the Medical Council under its disciplinary authority; a claim against a private hospital also concerns licensing and institutional oversight; a dispute about compensation may reach civil proceedings. The division protects different functions, but is difficult for a patient who does not know what remedy each pathway can provide.

An accessible system should begin with a single information gateway that triages the approach without requiring the person to choose a statutory provision. A representative explains whether the request concerns stopping a risk, obtaining a record, professional review, or compensation, and transfers it to the appropriate body with consent. A situation in which every body closes the case because the problem partly belongs to another body should be prevented.

A disciplinary proceeding protects professional standards, but does not always return money, treatment, or a rapid answer to the patient. An institutional complaint can correct service, but does not replace independent review when management is involved. A lawsuit may compensate, but it is expensive and slow. Explaining these differences in advance prevents false expectations and allows several pathways to be used when they complement one another.

The comparison with Israel sharpens the need for a simple map of redress and a duty to transfer matters among bodies. Multiple addresses are not a problem when responsibility for navigation exists; they become a harm when the patient is repeatedly sent back to start from the beginning.

Traditional and Complementary Medicine: Choice, Safety, and Licensing

In Thailand and Malaysia, traditional healing practices, herbal products, and complementary services exist alongside biomedical medicine. Their popularity alone does not prove effectiveness and does not justify automatic dismissal by the clinical team. Patients' rights require room for a conversation that does not mock belief or preference, while also requiring reliable information about risk, evidence, and interaction with medical treatment.

Patients sometimes conceal use of an herb or traditional practitioner because they fear criticism. Concealment can create risk during anesthesia, pregnancy, or treatment with medicines. A neutral question - what else are you taking or doing to treat the condition? - improves safety more than a blanket prohibition. The aim is to understand dose, source, frequency, and expectation and to build a plan that can realistically be followed.

Licensing should match the level of risk. Manual therapy, an herbal product, and an invasive procedure do not require the same framework. Training, advertising rules, prohibition of misleading claims, documentation, and referral to emergency medicine when warning signs appear should be established. A product sold as 'natural' requires quality control because an unknown source, contamination, or variable concentration impairs the ability to give meaningful consent.

Institutional integration does not mean granting approval to every tradition. It allows the system to define what can be offered, what remains experimental, and what is prohibited because of risk. In Israel, where patients also use complementary services, the lesson is to create a respectful documented conversation and connect regulation, pharmacy, and adverse-event reporting. Cultural choice is preserved when it rests on information and is not exploited by irresponsible marketing.

Medication Ingredients, Faith, and Transparency

In a multireligious system, a patient may attach importance to the source of a medication ingredient, the manufacturing process, or the route of administration. The question is not whether staff agree with the religious importance, but whether the information is material to the person's choice. Ignoring it can lead to later refusal or irregular use; an unsupported assurance can damage trust.

Physicians and pharmacists do not need to know every religious position in advance. They need to ask what matters to the patient, check reliable information, and state what is known and what is not. When an equivalent alternative exists, it can be offered. When there is no alternative and treatment is urgent, the risk should be explained, spiritual consultation allowed if time permits, and a competent decision respected.

Product labeling and an institutional information database can reduce the need to restart every inquiry, but they must be updated and must not turn a religious label into a medical verdict. Approval by a particular body does not establish suitability for every person, and absence of approval is not necessarily proof of prohibition. Transparency should present facts rather than decide on behalf of the patient.

The issue is relevant beyond Malaysia and beyond one religion. In Israel too, preferences concern kashrut, fasting, animal-derived ingredients, and timing of treatment. A procedure connecting pharmacy, the clinical team, and spiritual consultation can prevent conflict and preserve safety without turning faith into a stereotype.

Four Asian Countries - Four Rights Focal Points

Country	Systemic Basis	Typical Tension	Central Lesson
China	Expanded coverage, large hospitals, and digitization	Workload, incentives, and trust in information	Connect rights to transparency and primary care
Japan	Universal insurance, provider choice, and	Fragmentation of care and family	Coordination and advance planning are

Country	Systemic Basis	Typical Tension	Central Lesson
	an ageing system	burden	practical rights
Thailand	Three public schemes and rights-protection mechanisms	Access disparities and implementation of end-of-life directives	An administrative address and early conversation strengthen realization
Malaysia	Public-private system and multireligious society	Availability gaps and integration of family and faith	A uniform standard with individual adaptation and clear redress

The Asian chapter sharpens the idea of relational autonomy: a decision can remain autonomous within family, faith, or community, provided that the involvement was chosen by the person and does not replace the person's voice. For Israel, the lesson is to clarify in every encounter who is wanted in the conversation and what boundary of assistance the patient requests.

Chapter Thirteen: Africa - Nigeria and South Africa

Opening Dilemma

In a district where the number of dialysis stations is limited, a clinical team must choose among patients. The decision is difficult even when the criteria are professional. A threshold based on expected benefit may be justified, but it must be clear and must avoid hidden preference for those with money, connections, or the ability to arrive on time. The decision-making committee should include medical and ethical expertise, document its reasons, and allow review of exceptional cases. The physician at the bedside should not bear alone a decision that arises from a public shortage. The scenario shows that fair allocation is not merely a formula. A criterion such as 'ability to adhere' may discriminate against a person who lives far away or cannot miss work.

Legal equality begins where historical inequality is not denied.

Nigeria and South Africa illustrate two different challenges: building coverage and accountability in a resource-poor federal system, and realizing a strong constitutional right within a society that carries the legacy of apartheid and inequality.

1. Post-Colonialism and Health as Justice

African health systems were shaped by colonialism, borders, concentration of services in cities, and scarcity; rights must therefore be examined against a history of unequal distribution. Historically, colonial services often focused on particular populations, trade, and labor. After independence, states were required to expand services rapidly to villages and a growing population.

Within the service system, workforce shortages, migration of health professionals, weak infrastructure, and out-of-pocket payment limit realization of rights. Community and family play a major role where the state does not reach. For example, a right to maternal care is not meaningful when the clinic is distant, the road is impassable, and no staff are present at night. The barrier is not consent but the very existence of a service.

At the same time, applying the same immediate benchmark used for a wealthy country may be unfair. Scarcity, however, must not be used as an excuse for discrimination, corruption, or neglect of core services. Israel does not face scarcity on the same scale, but history shows that allocating resources according to political power preserves disparities. The periphery requires affirmative investment.

The right to health requires prioritizing primary care, water, sanitation, maternal health, and vaccination alongside institution-building. Justice is not only advanced technology.

2. Nigeria: Federalism, Out-of-Pocket Payment, and Expanding Insurance

Key sources: Nigeria National Health Act, 2014; NHIA Act, 2022.

Nigeria contends with a fragmented federal system and high out-of-pocket spending while newer legislation seeks to make insurance and a basic benefit package more accessible. Historically, the National Health Act of 2014 and the creation of basic financing mechanisms attempted to strengthen primary care. The National Health Insurance Authority Act of 2022 advanced broader mandatory coverage.

In clinical reality, the division of authority among the federation, states, and local governments makes uniformity difficult. Infrastructure and staffing vary greatly, and the private market fills gaps for those who can pay. A family required to pay in advance for emergency treatment may delay seeking care. Even when the law declares a basic package, a financing mechanism and transfer to a functioning facility are conditions for realizing it.

Mandatory insurance can expand solidarity but is difficult to implement in a largely informal labor market. Collection, registration, and trust in government are part of the challenge. Israel achieved near-universal registration through residency and health funds. This highlights the importance of a simple administrative mechanism, not only an abstract right.

Gradual expansion should guarantee a clearly defined package, subsidies for people in poverty, payment to providers, and quality oversight. An insurance card without a service is an empty promise.

A Responsibility Matrix in a Federal System

When authority is divided among levels of government, every essential service should specify who sets the standard, who finances it, who recruits staff, and who responds when the service is missing. Central government can define a basic package and equality rules; states can be responsible for planning and procurement; and local government for access, identifying barriers, and referral. From the person's perspective these are not three separate services, so a request should be received at one point even when its handling passes among authorities.

Budget transfers should be linked both to need and to performance, without punishing a population because its authority is weak. District-level indicators - medicine availability, staffing, referral time, and out-of-pocket spending - make it possible to identify where responsibility breaks down. Such a mechanism is relevant to Israel as well, where the state, health funds, hospitals, and local authorities each hold part of the pathway. Clarifying responsibility is not additional bureaucracy; it prevents a situation in which every body fulfills its narrow duty while the patient is left without a complete service.

3. South Africa: Section 27 and Progressive Realization

Key source: Constitution of South Africa, 1996, s. 27.

The South African Constitution anchors a right of access to health-care services and requires reasonable measures toward progressive realization, while prohibiting the refusal of emergency medical treatment. The 1996 Constitution was born after apartheid and sought to correct racially unequal allocation of resources. The National Health Act created a framework for a more unified system.

When the principle is translated into practice, a public sector serves most of the population with limited resources, while a developed private sector serves a minority. This gap is central to understanding the right. In the Treatment Action Campaign case, for example, the Court required the state to remove unreasonable restrictions on a medicine used to prevent mother-to-child transmission of HIV. The judgment emphasized reasonableness and the existence of a public program (Minister of Health v. Treatment Action Campaign (No. 2), 2002).

Courts nevertheless remain cautious about setting budgets, but they can examine whether policy includes vulnerable groups and whether restrictions are reasoned. This is an intermediate model between judicial abstention and direct management. Israel has no parallel constitutional clause, but the reasonableness model can enrich review of the benefits basket, waiting times, and disparities without turning a judge into a hospital manager.

The state should be required to present a plan, targets, priority for vulnerable groups, and a public explanation. Progressive realization is not a license for indefinite delay.

4. Rights, Scarcity, and Fair Allocation

In Africa, a central question is how to define a core of rights where resources are extremely limited, and how to prevent scarcity from becoming systematic harm to weaker regions and groups. Historically, global health programs sometimes focused on a single disease, producing important successes alongside parallel systems. Epidemics demonstrated the need to strengthen the system as a whole.

From an organizational perspective, an external donation may bring a medicine but may not fund staff, a laboratory, or the supply chain. Rights require enduring institutional capacity. A clinic that has an HIV program but no treatment for hypertension illustrates a distortion of priorities. A person is not a collection of separate projects.

In translating the principle into practice, defining a basic package may appear restrictive, but it can guarantee an equal minimum. It should be updated, evidence-based, and open to the public. Israel's Health Basket Committee is an example of a relatively visible allocation mechanism. Public representation, reason-giving, and transparency about equality considerations can be strengthened within it.

Fair allocation requires criteria, data, an appeal mechanism, and protection against corruption. Even a difficult decision can be legitimate when the process is proper.

5. Lessons for Israel: Affirmative Investment and Public Accountability

The African comparison reminds us that equality is not identical distribution, but greater investment where history, distance, and poverty create greater need. Historically, correcting inequality requires a shift from a formally neutral principle to disparity-oriented planning. Policy that does not see history preserves it.

Within the system itself, population-based budgeting alone may be insufficient for an area with high morbidity, workforce shortages, and high operating costs. A funding formula should weight need. A peripheral clinic, for example, may require workforce incentives, transport, and extended hours. Giving it the same per-capita budget as a central area is not necessarily equal.

Affirmative investment nevertheless generates opposition from those who fear losing resources. Transparency about data and objectives is essential to legitimacy. In Israel, disparities among Arab and Jewish localities and among the north, south, and center require binding targets. The Patients' Rights Law should be read together with distributive policy.

A rights-and-access indicator should be published by region, budgets should be linked to identified gaps, and progress in closing them should be reported. Public accountability is measured by outcomes, not merely by allocations.

Justice Under Scarcity: Progressive Realization of the Right

Scarcity does not absolve the state of responsibility, but it requires priorities that can be explained, reviewed, and appealed. This section focuses on transparency in allocation, the supply chain, inter-district disparities, and the ability to demonstrate measurable progress over time.

Scarcity exists, but it is not neutral: hospitals, specialists, and infrastructure were concentrated in particular regions and populations, and that gap continues to matter even after the law changes. Poor service is therefore not a natural condition merely because it has lasted for years. Progressive realization requires direction: the gap should narrow, not merely be managed. In Nigeria, responsibility is divided among levels of government; this fragmentation can enable local adaptation but can also create ambiguity. A medicine is missing from a clinic, and every actor refers the patient to another level. At the beginning of any financing arrangement, it should already be clear what will remain when the funding ends and who will bear the cost. A community may monitor and report; it should not have to finance from its own resources a service that the state has undertaken to provide. Regulation and training must address the movement of professionals, not only their total number. Even a relatively well-resourced system can create public scarcity if incentives pull workers into another sector. The right requires examining the result of distribution, not only the total amount of national expenditure.

Hard Allocation Decisions and Judicial Review

When the number of dialysis places is smaller than the need, every decision excludes someone whose condition may deteriorate. A court can examine whether criteria were published, applied consistently, and based on relevant medical information; it is poorly placed to decide directly who should receive treatment without seeing the full budgetary picture.

For that reason, an important remedy may be to require the system to give reasons, allow a rapid appeal, and publish a plan for expanding capacity. Such review does not eliminate scarcity, but it prevents scarcity from becoming an arbitrary or discriminatory decision.

Primary Care, Workforce, and Procurement: Primary care is a central tool for reducing disparities in maternal health, child health, and chronic disease. Constructing a building is not enough if there are no staff, medicines, or referral pathway. Days and hours of actual operation should be measured, not only the number of facilities. Procurement and inventory data are therefore rights indicators. Publishing them, protecting whistleblowers, and enabling community oversight are not governance issues separate from health; they determine whether a medicine reaches a person's hand. Workforce shortages are also shaped by internal and international migration. Wealthier countries and regions benefit from professionals trained elsewhere. The solution is not to prohibit movement, but to invest in training, working conditions, career pathways, and support for peripheral areas. Task-sharing with nurses and community health workers can expand access, but it must be accompanied by training, authority, and supervision. Transferring responsibility to a less senior worker without resources is not innovation; it is risk transfer. Traditional healers remain a major point of contact in some communities. Ignoring them does not prevent their use and may delay referral. Referral and education mechanisms can be built, warning signs identified, and boundaries maintained against harmful practices. Cooperation does not mean treating every method as equivalent; it means using existing reality to protect people. As in intercultural health, the community can help shape the pathway while the standard of safety and the individual's right remain intact.

Measurable Progressive Realization: Improvement in the average is not enough if the gap widens. Every target needs a date and a funding source. When a target is not achieved, the state should explain what changed and what correction will follow. Progressive realization then becomes a testable commitment rather than a slogan. It is necessary to examine not only how much users paid, but also who refrained from seeking care. Household surveys, debt data, and interviews can reveal foregone care that never appears in the medical record. If a free public service requires an expensive trip and a lost workday, its cost is not zero. An equitable policy should address indirect costs as well. The lesson for Israel is not to compare the depth of scarcity, but to understand that accumulated disparity can become entrenched even in a wealthier system. Beds, specialists, transportation, and availability should be measured according to practical access rather than formal coverage alone.

Workforce and Professional Migration

Nigeria and South Africa train professionals, some of whom move to other countries or to the private sector. The result is shortage precisely in weaker areas. Restricting migration is not a fair solution; what is needed are pay, working conditions, safety, and a professional pathway that makes staying possible. Financial incentives alone are insufficient if there is no equipment, housing, or education for families. Policy should monitor distribution and retention, not only the number of graduates. Task redistribution can expand services when it is accompanied by training, supervision, and referral. Nurses, community workers, and pharmacists can assume additional functions without lowering quality. Expanded scope must not be used as a substitute for investment. Patients should know who is treating them and what that person's training is. Clinical accountability and support must be clear, especially where the specialist is distant.

Private Services Amid Public Scarcity

South Africa has a developed private system alongside an overloaded public one. The disparity is not only in insurance but also in workforce, equipment, and time. Reform should examine how private resources can be integrated without drawing still more capacity away from the public sector. Contracting with a private provider may shorten a queue, but it requires rules on price, quality, and oversight. If the public pays, data and accountability should remain public. In Nigeria, high direct expenditure can cause a family to sell assets or forgo care. Expanding insurance must guarantee a clear package and an appeal mechanism. Registration alone is not coverage if the clinic still demands additional payment or lacks the medicine. Household surveys, mystery visits, and receipt audits can reveal the gap. Planning must include the informal sector, where many people work without an employer deducting contributions.

Trust After Institutional Harm: A general message that a service is open to everyone does not erase history. Consistent presence, representation within the workforce, and a response to complaints are required. When a community leader

cooperates, it is important to preserve voices that do not identify with that leader as well. Trust is not a short campaign but the result of encounters in which promises are kept. Research and public health should avoid language that blames a community for low adherence. The question should be whether the service is accessible, safe, and respectful. Rumors may arise from misinformation, but also from real experience. Dialogue makes it possible both to correct facts and to discover failures. Local teams need up-to-date information and the ability to acknowledge uncertainty. Credibility does not require an answer to everything, but honesty about what is known and what will be checked.

Constitutional Rights and Group Remedies

A service failure may affect an entire community, so an individual claim is sometimes insufficient. Structural orders, monitoring, and reporting can require a corrective program. A court should receive information on implementation rather than accept a promise alone. Public-interest organizations help maintain continuity. At the same time, prolonged litigation can become detached from the field; involving workers and residents in the corrective plan connects judgment with implementation. A group remedy should avoid overly detailed instructions that do not fit management. The court can set a target, transparency requirements, and a duty to present alternatives while leaving professionals to choose the means. Such review respects the government's role while requiring accountability. The right does not promise everything immediately; it prohibits indifference and requires reasonable progress.

Communicable Diseases and Individual Rights

Tuberculosis, HIV, and epidemics sharpen the tension between privacy and public health. Isolation, surveillance, and reporting may be justified, but they should be proportionate, limited, and accompanied by support. A person who cannot work or reach a clinic will not comply merely because an instruction was issued. Food, transport, and protection from stigma are part of the intervention. Coercion without support may deter people from testing and undermine the public objective. Consent to tests and disclosure of results require privacy even under conditions of scarcity. A crowded clinic can use appointment planning, a private conversation area, and simple measures to reduce exposure. Community participation can help adapt messages and reduce fear, but it does not authorize disclosure of personal information to a local leader. The balance between community trust and individual confidentiality should be explicit. The right to public health does not abolish the human rights it seeks to protect.

The Supply Chain as a Practical Right

A rural clinic has a skilled team, but an essential medicine does not arrive for weeks. From the patient's perspective, the distinction among a budget failure, tender problem, warehouse issue, or transport breakdown does not change the result. One accountable address is therefore needed that holds a complete picture of inventory and alternatives.

A monitoring system should identify an expected shortage before the shelf is empty, publish a clinical alternative, and document transfers among districts. When there is no substitute, priority rules and an explanation to patients should be defined. Data on stock-out days, emergency prices, and supply time make it possible to distinguish an unforeseeable crisis from a recurring management failure.

The case illustrates that progressive realization is measured in logistics as well. A constitutional right loses meaning when procurement, transport, and inter-authority responsibility do not function.

Community Insurance and the Risk of Exclusion

Community insurance schemes can pool resources where national coverage is partial, but a small risk pool is vulnerable to expensive illness and economic crisis. When enrollment is voluntary, younger and healthier people may remain outside and the fund struggles to finance those who are ill. When the contribution is uniform, people in poverty may be excluded.

A stable solution requires public subsidy, broad pooling, and rules that prevent refusal based on medical condition. The community can participate in management and oversight, but it should not carry alone a risk the state is able to spread. Transparency about the package, payment times, and appeals is essential so that insurance does not become an unrealizable promise.

For Israel, the implication is that supplementary or local insurance should also be evaluated by who remains outside it, not only by the services offered to those who are insured.

Climate, Epidemics, and System Resilience

Climate change increases heat stress, infectious disease, and damage to infrastructure. In regions where the system already lacks staff and inventory, an extreme event displaces routine services and deepens disparities. The right to health therefore includes resilience: water, electricity, cold chains, emergency inventory, and a plan for continuing chronic care.

Emergency planning should identify who depends on dialysis, oxygen, refrigerated medicines, or transport. Such a list is sensitive and requires privacy protection, but without it evacuation and supply become arbitrary. A local community can help identify needs and communicate, provided the state supplies resources and authority.

After the crisis, the system should examine who lost treatment and why. Reopening the clinic does not necessarily mean a return to normal if patients have been lost to follow-up.

Joint Procurement and Transparency: Countries or districts with limited purchasing power may pay higher prices and suffer unstable supply. Joint procurement can improve terms, but it requires reliable needs data, contracts that define supply times, and a mechanism for allocating inventory during shortages.

Deviations, penalties, and relationships with suppliers should be published without disclosing unnecessary commercial secrets. Transparency reduces corruption and helps determine whether a shortage resulted from the global market or a local decision. Here too, the right is realized through an administrative mechanism that appears distant from the treatment room but determines what will be on the shelf.

Maternal Health and Childbirth Under Scarcity

Shortages of staff, blood, transport, and operating rooms make pregnancy and childbirth an acute test of the right to health. A woman may receive basic follow-up yet have no rapid route to a center capable of treating hemorrhage or preeclampsia. Emergency availability is part of the service, not an extra measured only by the number of clinics.

In a multilingual and culturally diverse system, consent should also be protected under pressure. A brief explanation, an available interpreter, and privacy are not luxuries. A companion or traditional midwife can provide support, but their presence should not be used to transfer the responsibility for explanation or to delay referral when risk increases.

Review of a severe maternal event should be confidential enough to support learning but connected to accountability. The entire chain should be examined: recognition of a warning sign, referral, transport, admission, blood supply, and postpartum response. Blaming a woman for arriving late may conceal a long journey, cost, or distrust created in an earlier encounter.

Israel can learn from the importance of a regional network: a consultation hub, transport, transfer standards, and drills among institutions. Rights in the delivery room also depend on what happened hours earlier in the community and on the ability to arrive in time.

Humanitarian Aid and Parallel Systems

In countries facing scarcity or crisis, humanitarian organizations sometimes operate alongside the public service. They can bring medicines, staff, and mobile clinics rapidly, but can also create a parallel system that is not connected to the record, referral pathway, or national planning. A patient benefits from a temporary service but may be left without continuity when the project ends.

Coordination should not turn an independent organization into a government arm, especially when it serves a population that does not trust the authorities. Common standards are nevertheless needed for safety, consent-based information transfer, disease reporting, and referral. The patient should be told who holds the record and what will happen after the team leaves.

External resources may deepen disparities if they concentrate in locations accessible to donors or on diseases that attract attention. Mapping needs with the community and local authority helps select regions and services according to harm rather than visibility. Publishing the budget and duration of activity allows the public to prepare for the end of the program.

The goal is a transition from dependence to strengthened local capacity: workforce training, supply chains, maintainable equipment, and a handover pathway. Success is not only the number of visits during the project, but how much service remains functional afterward. This is a test of responsibility toward patients who did not choose whether care would be provided by a public or temporary system.

Accountability Indicators in a System Facing Scarcity

Domain	Accountability Question	Possible Indicator	Response to Failure
Treatment allocation	Are the criteria consistent and explainable?	Admission disparities by region and group	Publication of reasons and rapid appeal
Medicines and procurement	Was the shortage foreseeable and managed in time?	Stock-out days and cost of alternatives	Supply plan and identified budget responsibility
Workforce	Where are professionals missing, and why?	Filled positions and turnover	Incentives, safety, and career pathway
Geographic access	Does the service exist in the person's real life?	Travel time and lost workdays	Mobile service, transport, or decentralization
Annual progress	Is the gap actually narrowing?	Disaggregated multi-year trend	Order, corrective plan, and public reporting

The African comparison places at its center the meaning of a right under conditions of persistent scarcity. The duty is not to make a promise that cannot be kept, but to establish visible priorities, monitor disparities, supply and workforce, and demonstrate progress. The lesson for Israel is to measure the pathway from budgeting to the practical ability to reach care.

Chapter Fourteen: Europe - Britain and Germany

Opening Dilemma

A patient in Britain is waiting for surgery and does not know whether she can transfer to another hospital. A patient in Germany receives a list of providers but struggles to understand which are available and of good quality. Both need mediation, not merely information. In Britain, the patient should be updated about time and alternatives; in Germany, the patient needs help using the available choice. If the process fails, each person needs an address that does not require knowledge of the institutional structure. The comparison shows that both too little choice and too much choice can be ineffective in different ways. A public dashboard can include waiting times, cancellations, access to complaints, safety incidents, and regional disparities. The data should be understandable, disaggregated, and accompanied by explanation.

Europe teaches that there is no single institutional route to solidarity, but every route requires rules, funding, and trust.

Britain and Germany represent two major forms of the medical welfare state: a tax-funded national service versus multi-fund social insurance. Both combine patients' rights with public and professional responsibility.

1. Europe and Patients' Rights as a Welfare-State Project

In Europe, patients' rights developed within broad public or social systems, so autonomy was linked from the outset to universality, quality, and solidarity. After the Second World War, national services and social insurance expanded. European conventions, case law, and data protection added a regional layer of rights.

Institutionally, countries differ in financing and provision, but most recognize broad access and public oversight. Debate is more often about waiting times, provider choice, and financing innovation than about coverage itself. The right to consent can be realized in a system without a bill at the point of service, yet queues and scarcity still limit choice. Solidarity does not abolish rationing.

A public service can nevertheless become bureaucratic; regulated competition can improve responsiveness but also create fragmentation. No model is immune. Israel inherited European influences in its health funds and social insurance. The comparison is particularly relevant to the tension between competing health funds and state oversight.

Individual rights should be combined with system indicators, and choice should be enabled without undermining planning. Responsibility for the service remains public even when the provider is not governmental.

2. Britain: The NHS, Care Free at the Point of Use, and a Constitution

Key source: Department of Health and Social Care, 2023.

The NHS is based on comprehensive service according to need rather than ability to pay, and the NHS Constitution brings together rights, pledges, and responsibilities of patients, the public, and staff. Historically, the service was established in 1948. The NHS Constitution was first published in 2009 and is supported by a duty on relevant bodies to have regard to it, although it largely consolidates rights that already existed.

Within the system, the Constitution includes rights to access, quality, dignity, consent, confidentiality, choice, and complaint, alongside staff rights and public responsibilities to use resources fairly. A patient, for example, is entitled to information about waiting times and to choice in certain circumstances. If waiting exceeds the applicable maximum, there are routes to request another provider, although implementation depends on capacity.

Even so, pledges that are not legal rights can create expectation without a remedy. The distinction between a right and a pledge in the Constitution seeks to be honest, but can also confuse. Israel can learn from concentrating rights and responsibilities in an accessible document and from including staff rights. Israeli law is more detailed in some fields but less explicit about the broader compact.

A complementary Israeli charter could clarify rights, responsibilities, and routes of enforcement in public language without replacing the law.

3. Germany: Mandatory Insurance and Corporatist Self-Governance

Key sources: WHO, 2019; European Observatory, 2020.

Germany guarantees mandatory insurance through statutory or private coverage and manages a large part of the system through bodies of insurers and providers operating within a legal framework. Historically, German social insurance has roots in the nineteenth century. The model developed into multiple statutory funds, regulated competition, and tariffs and benefits determined through self-governance processes.

In practice, most of the population is covered by statutory insurance and a smaller share by substitutive private insurance. Decisions on benefits and quality are made by joint bodies in which professional organizations and insurers have substantial power. Patients enjoy broad access to physicians but can encounter differences in availability between insurance types and significant bureaucratic complexity. Formal entitlement does not eliminate provider incentives.

The picture is more complex still: professional self-governance protects against day-to-day politicization and makes use of expertise, but it can be distant from the public and preserve the interests of powerful bodies. Israel's health funds and professional associations give its system some corporatist features as well. Meaningful patient representation is needed in decisions about quality and the benefits package.

Shared governance should include transparency, disclosure of conflicts of interest, and a public voice. Expertise is not a substitute for legitimacy.

Self-Governance: The Advantage of Expertise and the Test of Legitimacy

Joint bodies of insurers and providers can update technical rules relatively quickly and draw on knowledge from the field. Precisely because of their power, decisions about benefits, quality, or payment should also be understandable to people who are not members of the professional system. Publishing the agenda, a summary of evidence, conflicts of interest, and the reasons for the decision allows the public to see the values and compromises behind a rule that may appear purely technical.

Patient representation should not amount to a seat without resources. Effective representation requires access to information, professional advice, and time to respond before a decision is taken. After the decision, there should be a route for appeal and reassessment of its effect on availability and disparities between groups. This is an important lesson for Israel: the benefits of expertise and institutional negotiation can be preserved while still requiring public explanation and oversight of outcomes, not merely of procedural correctness.

4. Patients' Rights, Staff Responsibility, and Enforcement

European models emphasize that patients' rights exist alongside workers' rights, professional regulation, and complaint mechanisms that do not have to begin in court. Ombudsmen, regulators, quality bodies, and compensation mechanisms developed to resolve complaints and generate learning. Different countries balance tort litigation with administrative arrangements in different ways.

From an institutional perspective, a multi-channel approach makes it possible to choose among explanation, correction, discipline, and compensation. It reduces dependence on expensive litigation, but requires independence and authority. A complaint about disrespectful treatment, for example, can receive an organizational response even without medical injury. If the only mechanism is a lawsuit, most violations of dignity remain unaddressed.

Yet multiple bodies can also confuse. The patient needs one gateway that routes the complaint, and the worker needs to know that the process is fair and does not presume guilt. Israel has public inquiries mechanisms, the National Health Insurance complaints commissioner, and professional proceedings, but the system is fragmented. A rights map and a unified pathway could improve accessibility.

An independent contact point, clear timelines, and publication of anonymized decisions should be established. Learning must return to the field rather than remain in the file.

5. Lessons for Israel: A Charter of Rights and Responsibilities Alongside the Law

Europe offers Israel a complementary model: binding law alongside an accessible public document presenting rights, system commitments, and the mutual responsibilities of patients and staff. Historically, public charters can be updated and allow value-based discussion without reopening every statutory provision. They can respond relatively quickly to technology, privacy, and violence.

For an institution, a charter is insufficient without enforcement, but it can be a powerful educational and managerial tool. It clarifies who is responsible, what can be expected, and how a person can appeal. On entering an institution, a patient would receive not only a list of prohibitions but a short document explaining what the patient is entitled to, what is expected, how privacy is protected, and who can help in a dispute.

Responsibility discourse can, however, be misused to restrict care. It should be stated explicitly that the charter does not detract from urgent treatment or authorize punishment of a group. In Israel, a national charter could create a common language across health funds and hospitals, include staff safety, and connect the 1994 and 1996 laws.

The charter should be developed with patients, staff, organizations, and civil society, updated regularly, and measured in practice. In that way it becomes a tool rather than a poster.

Realization in a Welfare State: Waiting, Choice, and Complaint

Britain and Germany guarantee broad coverage through different institutions, but in both systems the right is tested by time, by the ability to understand the pathway, and by the existence of an address for complaints. This section focuses on the mediation and oversight mechanisms that allow a person to use the system rather than merely be entitled to it on paper.

Two Routes to the Same Public Promise: The British model creates basic equality and public trust but depends heavily on budget, workforce, and prioritization. When the queue grows, the patient is still entitled to know the urgency, when an examination is expected, and what alternatives exist. Universality is not a license for silence. If a waiting-time target is missed, the system should update the patient and permit review of priority. Such information is not a substitute for shortening the queue, but it prevents waiting from becoming a space without accountability. The German model's dispersion creates checks and provider choice but can make it harder for a person to know who has authority. Professional self-governance can adapt decisions to clinical reality, but it requires transparency and public oversight. When treatment is denied, the patient should not have to master the architecture of the system simply to know where to turn. A clear contact point can operate above fragmentation and allow institutions to resolve responsibilities behind the scenes. German patients' rights legislation consolidated rules on the treatment contract, information, consent, documentation, and burden of proof. This consolidation creates a clear language, but does not abolish the roles of insurers and providers. Both tools are useful when connected to a pathway, a timeframe, and responsibility. A document that does not tell a person what to do when a promise is breached may increase cynicism.

Managing the Queue as a Duty of Information and Fairness: Waiting time is not merely an efficiency indicator. It affects pain, risk, ability to work, and trust in the system. Institutional duties include publishing an estimated time, prioritizing according to medical need, updating the patient when circumstances change, and offering an alternative when the target exceeds what is reasonable.

Transparency does not guarantee a short queue, but it allows a person to understand where they stand in the pathway and to challenge an incorrect classification. Data should be published by region and group so that national averages do not conceal persistent disparities.

A Complaint That Moves Between Bodies Without Being Lost: In a multi-provider system, one complaint may involve a physician, a health fund, a hospital, and a financing body. The complainant should not have to know in advance who is responsible. One gateway receives the complaint, assigns a case owner, and transfers components to the relevant bodies while maintaining a shared timeline.

The response should distinguish between an individual solution and a system lesson. When the same failure recurs across different providers, the regulator should issue guidance or change an incentive rather than leave every complaint as a local case.

Solidarity and Workforce: Both systems face aging, workforce shortages, and digitization. Rights cannot be realized if there is no time for conversation or if appointments are repeatedly cancelled. Workforce policy is therefore part of rights policy. Recruitment alone is not enough; working conditions, training, and protection from burnout are also required. When staff cannot deliver the promise, frustration should not be directed only at them. Responsibility also lies in planning and budgeting. Patient responsibilities in service charters can include providing information, respecting staff, and using resources fairly. They must not be used to deny care to a person who behaved imperfectly or failed to follow an instruction. Responsibility is not symmetrical: the institution holds power, budget, and alternatives. When behavior endangers others, limits can be set and the mode of service changed, but essential care remains a duty. Properly framed responsibilities clarify expectations without turning a right into a reward for good behavior.

The General Practitioner as Guardian of Continuity: A gateway can coordinate care and prevent duplication, but it can also delay specialist access. Broad choice can accelerate access but fragment care. Every model therefore requires someone who holds the overall picture. In Britain, where general practitioners play a central role in navigating specialist services, the quality of the gateway is tested by its ability to update urgency and consolidate information returned from the referred service. In Germany, where patients often have broader direct mobility among specialists, the challenge is different: ensuring that results, treatment changes, and repeat prescriptions return to someone who maintains the overall picture and prevents duplicate testing. Incentives should therefore reward coordination, not only separate activity.

Electronic Records and European Trust

Expanding digital records can improve continuity, but sensitivity to privacy is high in Europe. A model that includes consent, the option to restrict, and documented access strengthens control. Excessive complexity can mean that people do not understand the settings. A short explanation and cautious defaults are preferable to a long document. Patients should be able to see who accessed their information and report unusual use. Information for research and public planning is important, but it should be distinguished from treatment. Secondary use should be protected, supervised, and explained. Refusal should not damage access to care. Where data are reliably anonymized, broader use may be justified, but zero risk should not be promised. Transparency about benefit, partners, and security enables public discussion rather than merely technical consent.

Medicine Shortages and Cross-Border Supply

Europe's medicine supply chain crosses countries, manufacturers, and distributors. A factory failure or export restriction can affect a patient who has no idea where the shortage originated. Early reporting, a shared inventory database, and agreement on clinical alternatives across systems are therefore needed.

Cross-border information sharing does not release the local body from responsibility for explaining to the patient what changed. Practical protection is a continuous chain: early identification, fair allocation, notification of staff and patients, and follow-up of those whose treatment must change.

Choosing Between Providers: Continuity During Transfer: The difference between a broad provider market and a coordinated pathway becomes especially clear when a patient moves between institutions or physicians. In Britain, moving between practices or regions requires assurance that the record and ongoing treatment are not interrupted; in Germany, more direct choice among specialists heightens the need to transfer results and define who renews prescriptions. A sound mechanism should guarantee continuity during the transition: an up-to-date clinical summary, transfer of tests, identification of a contact person, and an overlap period where a medicine or follow-up must not be interrupted. Choice is then measured not only by the number of providers but also by the quality of movement between them.

Workforce, Migration, and the Ethics of Recruitment

Britain and Germany rely heavily on professionals trained in other countries. Recruitment helps address shortages but raises questions about working conditions, recognition of qualifications, and effects on countries of origin. A system that speaks of rights should also protect migrant workers from discrimination and dependency. Training in professional language and organizational culture should be funded rather than imposed on the worker alone. Staff who feel that they belong and are safe are better able to explain decisions and set boundaries. Long-term planning should examine not only the number of posts but who stays, in which regions, and under what shift burden. Attrition is a quality indicator. When a department depends on overtime and constant replacement, the risk of rights violations increases. Publishing workforce data alongside waiting times helps reveal the relationship and avoids blaming staff. Solutions may include training, retention, task distribution, and technology, but every tool should be assessed for its effect on the patient relationship.

Continuity of Care When Moving Between Systems

A person who worked in Germany and returned to Britain needs to continue treatment begun with a specialist. The documents exist, but codes, medicine names, and the route to a specialist are different. Without a coordinating body, responsibility shifts to the patient and treatment may stop while the systems verify eligibility.

A transition pathway should include a clinical summary in an agreed format, temporary verification of coverage, and a receiving body that confirms continuation of treatment. The case shows that mobility and formal entitlement are not enough; the right is tested by whether a clinical decision can pass between institutions without starting again from zero.

The issue is especially acute in complex chronic care. A patient who moved from Germany to Britain receives a biologic medicine at fixed intervals, but the new framework requires different tests and local authorization before the next dose. A continuity pathway should include the indication, previous failed treatments, date of the last dose, safety results, and a bridging plan until the local specialist decides. Here the problem is not provider choice but preservation of clinical logic while responsibility moves. Without a temporary bridge, an administrative difference between systems can become an interruption in treatment that nobody intended.

Cross-Border Care in the European Union

A European patient may obtain treatment in another country when a service is not available within a reasonable time, but practical entitlement depends on authorization, reimbursement, translation, and follow-up after returning home. Incomplete information about costs or reimbursement conditions can make the right accessible only to those who can pay in advance.

A fair pathway should present local alternatives, expected waiting time, the amount to be reimbursed, and responsibility for complications. A medical summary should be sent in a format understandable to the receiving institution, and the local physician should receive results and the care plan. Otherwise cross-border treatment creates a gap in continuity.

The mechanism demonstrates that broad choice requires a coordination infrastructure. The mere ability to travel is not equality when language, money, and information determine who can use it.

An Independent Ombudsman

An ombudsman with institutional independence can examine a complaint without being part of the organization complained about. Its authority may include obtaining documents, hearing the parties, recommending compensation or change, and publishing reports. Its value lies not only in individual resolution but also in identifying systemic failures across institutions.

To preserve trust, response times, appeal options, and conflict-of-interest rules should be defined. The ombudsman does not replace the courts in serious cases, but offers a more accessible and rapid pathway. Publishing the implementation rate of recommendations is as important as publishing the number of complaints.

In Israel, such a model could connect complaints, safety, and quality without forcing the patient to choose the correct body in advance.

Patient Participation in Service Design

Britain and Germany have different mechanisms for public participation, but they face the same challenge: avoiding a situation in which one representative merely approves a plan that has already been decided. Meaningful participation begins before the solution is chosen, provides data, and clarifies which decisions remain open.

Patients can identify barriers that are invisible in professional indicators - a letter that is hard to understand, a time that does not fit public transport, or a transfer between call centers. Staff add information about workload and safety. Combining these voices does not eliminate professional responsibility; it improves the design of the pathway by which the service reaches the person.

After implementation, participants should be told what was adopted and what was not. Such feedback turns participation into an ongoing process rather than a public-relations event.

Health Technology Assessment and Patient Participation

Britain and Germany use institutional mechanisms to assess medicines and technologies before broad public funding. Decisions combine effectiveness, safety, cost, and sometimes added value compared with an alternative. The process protects public budgets, but may appear to the patient as a numerical decision that fails to see a rare disease or an individual need.

Patient participation can add information that is not captured in trials: effects on function, treatment burden, burden on family caregivers, and the value of a small improvement. Testimony does not replace comparative evidence, but it can help select relevant outcomes and identify costs that an economic model missed.

To reduce bias, relationships with manufacturers should be disclosed, different groups should be represented, and the process should explain how testimony affected the decision. A negative decision should include reasons, conditions for reconsideration, and a pathway for exceptional cases. Transparency does not guarantee agreement, but it makes review possible and allows new evidence to be brought forward.

For Israel, it is relevant to strengthen public participation in benefits-basket and technology deliberations without turning the process into a competition of dramatic stories. A fixed framework, an evidence document, and a reasoned response can connect budgetary justice with patient experience.

Two Welfare Systems - Three Tests of Use

The European comparison shifts the center of gravity from entitlement itself to responsibility within a welfare system:

waiting time, choice, complaint, self-governance, and the reasoning behind funding. For Israel, the lesson is that universality needs a mechanism that explains limits, allows review, and retains responsibility until a case is resolved or properly transferred.

Test	**Britain**	**Germany**	**Transferable Principle**
Waiting time	Public targets and centralized prioritization	Broader access to providers but variable availability	Updates, an alternative option, and priority according to risk
Provider choice	A significant gatekeeping role for the general practitioner	Self-governance and multiple funds and providers	A mediator who explains options rather than merely providing a list
Complaint	A local pathway followed by an external body	Complex professional and insurance contact points	One gateway that retains responsibility until an answer is given
Digital information	Linkage among public services	More decentralized systems	Clear authorization and documented access
Workforce	Dependence on international recruitment under pressure	Regional shortages and recognition of qualifications	Working conditions and recruitment ethics as part of rights

Part Five: Between Rights and Responsibility - Synthesis and Recommendations for the Future

The final part brings together the historical journey, Israeli law, and the international comparison. It does not seek to choose between the patient and the physician, but to reject the very framing in which the rights of one exist at the expense of the safety and dignity of the other. A worthy health system distributes responsibility among the state, the organization, the profession, and the public, and recognizes that rights require resources, culture, and mechanisms of correction.

Chapter Fifteen: Between Right and Responsibility - The Future of the Clinician-Patient Relationship

Opening Dilemma

Three hospitals introduce a discharge coordinator. After six months, documentation improves, but readmissions fall at only one site. Review shows that at the other two sites the coordinator lacked authority to book appointments or order equipment. Rather than scaling the model unchanged, management revises the coordinator's authority and continues the trial. The report publishes the gap as well as the achievement. This is what responsible learning looks like: a target, data, explanation, and correction. It does not require reform to succeed immediately, but neither does it allow reform to continue on prestige alone. The public and staff know what was learned, and expansion is conditioned on real capacity rather than a headline. Ultimately, the proposed program does not seek to add another bureaucratic layer above an already burdened system.

Benevolence without rights depends on the will of the powerful; rights without benevolence can become a cold procedure. Humane medicine needs both.

The next generation of patients' rights should move from a model focused on preventing harm to one focused on real capability: to understand, participate, receive care in time, and act in an environment that is safe for both patient and staff.

1. What Changed on the Journey from Benevolence to Rights

The historical journey reveals a consistent pattern: whenever medicine expanded its power through knowledge, institutions, research, financing, or technology, a mechanism became necessary to restrain that power and return a voice to the person. At first these were professional duties; later, law, participation, and corrective mechanisms were added. The layers do not cancel one another; they correct one another's weaknesses.

Failure does not always occur where a right is formulated. It may arise in a queue, in translation, in transfer of a record, in the absence of an address for appeal, or when a worker is left alone facing a demand they have no authority to resolve. We therefore need to track the pathway a person travels until the right can actually be used, and at the same time the conditions that allow staff to set boundaries and receive institutional backing.

This leads to the starting point for reform: neither a return to unilateral authority nor transfer of full responsibility to the patient, but supported autonomy within a system that openly states its limits. Every change should be assessed by the gap it addresses - information, access, accountability, remedy, or safety - and by the body that actually holds the means to correct it.

Success should be measured not by the number of forms, but by the proportion of people who understood, received care in time, felt respected, and knew how to appeal - and by the proportion of workers who returned home safely.

2. A Four-Layer Model for Realizing Rights

Realizing rights requires four layers at the same time: a legal norm, organizational design, professional capability, and public culture. Failure in one layer weakens the others. Many reforms have focused on only one layer - a new law, campaign, form, or security measure - and discovered that change does not endure without system-wide alignment.

In implementation, law defines the floor; the organization allocates time, space, and staff; the profession translates the principle into conversation and decision; and the public understands both the right and its limits. A right to an interpreter is not realized if there is no budget, if staff do not know how to order the service, if the interpreter arrives too late, or if the patient is afraid to use it (Gostin, 2014; Yamin, 2023).

In practice, dividing responsibility can turn into dispersing blame. Every right therefore needs an identifiable owner and a testable outcome, rather than a general statement that 'the system' is responsible. At the synthesis stage the principle is enough: there is no effective right without a clear address. The practical division of authority among bodies appears later in the implementation plan.

An implementation map should be built for every major provision of the law: process, responsible body, resource, indicator, complaint route, and correction. In this way the law becomes an operating system rather than only a normative document.

3. Proposed Reforms in Israel

The update required is not a wholesale replacement of the 1996 law, but a clear determination of which gaps require legal amendment and which result from poor design. Since the law was enacted, the information environment, modes of care, and the structure of relationships with families have changed, while the principles of dignity, consent, and confidentiality remain valid. Priorities should be set according to severity of harm, scope, and capacity for correction - not according to the newest technology or the latest public pressure.

Three prioritization tests can guide change: Is the right available at the time it is needed? Is responsibility identifiable, and can a decision be appealed? Is implementation possible without imposing an invisible task on an existing workforce? New technology should be judged by the same tests. A computerized recommendation system, for example, is not problematic merely because it is new, but when no person can explain the recommendation, review an exception, and take responsibility for the decision.

Additional regulation can deepen failure if it adds a form without authority, time, or resources. Before creating a new duty, existing duties should be mapped, duplicate reporting removed, and the possibility of achieving the outcome through process redesign examined. Only a gap that cannot be solved administratively - such as the independence of an oversight body or binding rules for algorithmic decisions that materially affect care - justifies legislative amendment.

Every proposal should define an outcome rather than only an action: what should change in patient experience, worker safety, and disparities between groups. The next section does not offer another list of promises; it offers an execution mechanism that connects each target to authority, budget, indicators, and stopping conditions.

Immediate Steps That Do Not Require Legislation

Within one year, every institution can be required to publish a plain-language map of rights and contact points, appoint an accountable person for complaint and appeal pathways, establish a procedure for interpreter-assisted conversations, and identify high-risk transitions after discharge. Responsibility for implementation lies with institutional and health-fund management under Ministry of Health oversight. Success should be measured by time to response, the proportion of patients who know where to turn, use of professional interpretation, and completion of follow-up actions set at discharge. These steps do not create new rights; they make existing rights visible and accessible.

Organizational and Budgetary Reforms

In the medium term, protected time should be allocated for complex conversations, coordination roles should be expanded for high-risk patients, a permanent support system should be available to workers after violence, and complaint, safety, and continuity data should be connected. The Ministry of Health should set standards, while funding and implementation are divided among the state, health funds, and hospitals according to control of the resource. Indicators should not be limited to the number of positions or training sessions, but include reductions in waiting and access disparities, fewer preventable readmissions, better understanding of care plans, and a higher proportion of workers reporting that they received backing. Published data should be disaggregated and avoid simplistic ranking of institutions serving different populations.

Long-Term Legislative Amendments

Future legislation should address areas where administrative procedure is insufficient: independence and authority of a rights commission, rules governing material uses of artificial intelligence, a right to explanation of automated decisions, protection of secondary-use data, and binding timelines where delay makes an appeal meaningless. It may also be appropriate to require anonymized publication of the principles behind ethics-committee decisions and of system lessons. The Knesset would set the framework, the Ministry of Health would issue implementation rules, and an independent body would assess implementation. Success would be measured by the ability to obtain correction in time, reduced unjustified variation among institutions, and the proportion of systemic recommendations actually implemented - not by the number of proceedings opened.

4. A New Compact Between Patients and Staff

The way to reduce conflict is not to weaken one side but to build a compact based on truth, boundaries, correction, and support. Trust is not obedience; it is a willingness to place vulnerability in a worthy system. Historically, the Hippocratic compact was relatively one-sided; the consumer contract is bilateral but market-oriented. A public compact adds the responsibility of the state and the interests of other patients.

In practice, the organization commits to information, reasonable time, equality, privacy, and safety. The patient commits to providing information, respecting workers and others, and using appeal pathways. The worker commits to professionalism and transparency. When failure occurs, the compact is tested: Does the institution disclose, apologize, and correct? Does the family have a route to be heard? Does the worker receive a fair process and support?

A compact is not full symmetry. The patient is vulnerable and dependent, so the institution carries a heightened duty. Patient responsibility is not a condition for dignity or urgent care. In Israel, the language of a compact fits a tradition of mutual responsibility, but it must be universal and must not depend on identity, connections, or contribution to the state.

The compact should be embedded in education, signage, complaint processes, and management indicators. A document without consistent behavior will deepen cynicism.

5. Conclusion: Preserving the Human Within the System

Patients' rights are intended to protect the human being where fear, knowledge, and technology create asymmetries of power. Protecting staff serves the same goal: enabling care without fear and humiliation. From the ancient healer to the digital hospital, the ill body remains vulnerable and knowledge remains unequal. The modern innovation is that this inequality does not grant a license to control.

At the system level, a worthy system does not promise that every wish will be fulfilled or every disease cured. It promises that decisions will be made fairly, that information will not be withheld without justification, and that pain will not make a person invisible. The decisive moment may be small: a staff member closes a curtain, explains again, calls an interpreter, or honestly says that no bed is available and when an update will come. In that moment, the law acquires a body.

At the same time, a system cannot be built on the daily heroism of workers. Humane gestures require standards, time, management, and funding; otherwise they erode. Israel's challenge is to preserve excellence and initiative while moving from a culture of improvisation to planned rights. This is not a criticism of medicine's sense of mission; it is a way to protect it.

There is no need to choose between benevolence and rights. Benevolence adds compassion beyond the minimum; rights ensure that the minimum does not depend on benevolence. Their combination is the foundation of democratic medicine.

A National Program: Implementing the Clinician-Patient Compact

The national execution mechanism connects allocation of authority, budgeting, baseline indicators, risk management, independent evaluation, and orderly transfer between administrations and governments. The test is not the number of declarations but the ability to demonstrate stable change over time.

Governance, Targets, and Accountability

Before launching reform, the current state should be measured: waiting times, quality of consent, rate of repeated complaints, violence, worker absences, and regional disparities. A target without a baseline makes it possible to declare success even when nothing changed. Indicators should be defined uniformly but adapted to service type so that an emergency department is not compared mechanically with a scheduled clinic.

Every target should have a desired value, a timeframe, and a responsible owner. Alongside each quantitative indicator there should be an experiential measure examining whether the public knows the pathway, trusts it, and receives an understandable response.

A Binding Map of Authority.

Reform stalls when the Ministry of Health, health funds, hospitals, and local authorities assume that someone else is responsible. An authority map should define who sets the standard, who funds it, who implements it, who collects data, and who is authorized to correct a deviation. Each initiative should have one lead body even when implementation is shared.

The map should be published for the public and staff in plain language. People can then know where to turn and who is required to respond, and responsibility does not dissolve among committees.

Resources, Workforce, and Contracting

Every target should have a budget line or an explanation of how it will be financed from existing resources. One-time costs, such as an information system, should be distinguished from recurring costs for staff, translation, or worker support. A temporarily funded pilot is not proof that a national service can be sustained for years.

The budget report should also present the cost of inaction: repeat admissions, claims, absences, and lost time. Connecting cost with outcome allows priorities to be selected rather than presenting every component as an isolated obligation.

Training and support in routine work.

A new procedure does not change behavior if workers do not receive time, tools, and feedback. Training should be based on real-world scenarios, practice, and incident analysis rather than only a presentation. Managers should receive tools to examine whether a process is feasible under peak workload and to redesign work allocation accordingly.

During implementation, a professional helpdesk should answer questions and collect difficulties from departments. Rapid correction of a form or process is preferable to insisting on wording that does not work.

Pilot, Evaluation, and Stopping Conditions

Every initiative should have a risk map: privacy harm, transfer of burden to another worker, longer queues, patient labeling, or creation of a complaint channel without real power. Each risk should have an early warning sign and a preventive action. Reform is then assessed not only by its intended benefit but also by possible harm.

An adverse event during a pilot should not automatically cancel the initiative. It should be examined to distinguish a correctable failure from a fundamental design flaw.

Independent evaluation and learning across institutions.

The body responsible for implementation should not be the only body evaluating its own success. An independent evaluation team should receive access to data, interview workers and patients, and publish findings even when they are uncomfortable. Independence does not mean detachment: evaluators should work with institutions to understand context, but should not be subordinate to management targets.

Institutions should share failures and corrections as well as successes. Such learning requires protection against using reports for simplistic rankings or punishment; otherwise every organization will present only achievements.

Phased expansion and stopping conditions.

A pilot should expand only if it met pre-specified conditions: improved outcomes, no significant harm, sustainable financing, and reasonable satisfaction among users and workers. If results are mixed, one component can be expanded while another is modified. There is no need to choose between total success and total failure.

Stopping or pause conditions should also be defined. Such a mechanism protects against continuing investment in an initiative that does not work merely because it has already been announced.

Continuity across administrations and governments.

A multi-year program needs institutional memory. Every change in leadership should be accompanied by a status document: decisions, budget, data, risks, and open commitments. Permanent professional office-holders should preserve continuity even when political priorities change.

Policy changes should remain possible, but they should require public reasons and assessment of their effect on initiatives already underway. This reduces the pattern in which pilots are abandoned and restarted without learning.

Equality and Public Participation

Public participation is not an opening ceremony. Representatives of patients, families, and workers should participate in defining indicators, reviewing information materials, and interpreting results. Participants should be diverse and given data and time; otherwise participation becomes a ritual of approval.

When a professional recommendation does not adopt a public position, it should explain why. Explanation preserves trust and clarifies that participation is neither a veto right nor decoration.

The Five-Year Test.

After five years, reform should be assessed on three dimensions: whether rights are better understood and realized, whether working conditions and safety improved, and whether disparities among groups and regions narrowed. Evaluation should also examine unintended costs and effects on services that were not the original focus.

The conclusion may be continuation, substantial redesign, or termination of a component. Responsible reform does not commit forever to its first wording; it commits to measuring, explaining, and correcting.

Program Management Unit.

Large-scale reform needs a small permanent unit that coordinates timelines, dependencies among initiatives, and open decisions. The unit does not replace office-holders in organizations; it ensures that every task is linked to an accountable owner, budget, and indicator, and that change in one area does not create failure in another.

Once a month, initiatives should be reviewed against milestones rather than narrative reports. Barriers should be escalated to the level capable of resolving them, and a decision log should be preserved to prevent the same arguments from recurring after leadership changes. The unit should publish a public summary that protects sensitive information while showing progress and delays.

To avoid becoming another bureaucratic layer, the unit's authority should be limited to coordination, oversight, and escalation. Professional and managerial responsibility should remain where the service is delivered.

Equality Impact Assessment.

Every initiative should be assessed in advance for its effect on peripheral areas, language, disability, age, and economic status. A digital service may shorten queues for most people while excluding those without a device; a detailed form may improve documentation while burdening people who struggle to read. Equality impact assessment identifies such effects before expansion.

Each risk should have an accommodation: a non-digital route, translation, additional time, or reinforcement in a weaker region. After implementation, disaggregated data should be published while protecting privacy. A gap that remains unchanged should require modification, not merely explanation.

Equality does not require an identical process for everyone. It requires that different pathways lead to a similarly real opportunity to understand, choose, and receive service.

Information Infrastructure and Digital Rights

Rights and continuity depend on the ability to transfer information among health funds, hospitals, and services. A new system should not create yet another database that does not communicate with existing ones. Standards, patient identity, permissions, access logs, and the ability to correct errors should be defined. Patients should be able to see who viewed their information and what was transferred.

Interoperability is not only a technical issue. The meaning of fields, responsibility for updates, and what happens when two records conflict must be agreed. Clinical, legal, and technological teams should work together, and patient representatives should test whether the interface is understandable and useful.

During transition, dual systems should be operated carefully and information loss prevented. A single launch date without phased testing can turn the reform itself into a safety risk.

Contracting and Procurement.

Parts of reform will be performed by vendors: information systems, translation, call centers, and training. Contracts should define not only outputs but outcomes, availability, privacy, and transfer of knowledge to the public system. A vendor that hoards data or controls code that cannot be transferred creates long-term dependency.

A tender should include a trial period, accessibility testing, and an exit clause if the service fails to meet requirements. Criteria and conflicts of interest should be published, and low price should not be achieved by overloading workers or reducing patient support.

At the end of a contract, data, documentation, and the ability to continue the service should remain with the public body.

Workforce Strategy.

Rights should not be implemented by adding tasks to the same number of workers. Roles, required time, and competencies should be mapped: who explains, who coordinates transition, who answers a complaint, and who analyzes data. Some work can be integrated into an existing role, while other work requires a new position or redistribution.

The strategy should include recruitment, retention, and training, but also removal of tasks that do not add value. Automation can reduce data entry provided it does not create additional checking or damage the relationship. Workforce indicators should include turnover, burnout, and ability to take breaks, not only the number of posts.

Workers should participate in process design. A solution that does not fit peak workload will be bypassed even if it looks excellent in a procedure manual.

Review and Sunset Clauses.

When an experimental component receives legal authorization, a date should be set at which the authority itself expires unless a new decision is made. This differs from stopping an operational pilot: it requires the legislature or regulator to revisit the justification, the effect on rights, and alternatives that have emerged since enactment.

Extension should require a public report and a reasoned decision, not occur by silence. Duties shown to be beneficial can become permanent arrangements; exceptional powers that were unused or caused harm should expire. This prevents temporary mechanisms from accumulating into permanent ones without debate.

The system thereby learns to view change as an ongoing process rather than a one-time legislative event.

A Joint Council of Patients and Workers.

A national program needs a body in which service experience and work experience are heard at the same table. A joint council does not replace a regulator or professional committee; its role is to identify early when a solution benefits one group while transferring the cost to another. For example, a more accessible public inquiry channel can create an impossible workload if staffing, triage, and response times are not defined.

Council members should be selected from varied regions, professions, ages, languages, and health conditions. Representation is not measured only by the number of seats: participants need materials in advance, support in understanding data, and reasonable compensation for their time. Conflicts of interest should be disclosed and terms limited so that representation does not become a closed profession.

The council should review forms, indicators, and pilot results and be able to demand a reasoned response. It should not have a veto over clinical or budgetary decisions, but rejection of its recommendation should be published with an explanation. Such a mechanism gives participation weight without obscuring who bears final responsibility.

Once a year, the council's own work should also be reviewed: which changes followed its recommendations, which groups were not heard, and whether discussion drifted away from the field. Public participation that also examines itself is less likely to become a symbol without influence.

Public Reporting and Learning

An annual report should bring together a limited set of national indicators: understanding of information, waiting times, complaints, continuity, violence, burnout, and disparities. Each number should be accompanied by a definition, data source, and any change in measurement method. An institution should not present a fall in complaints as success without checking whether the public is still using the channel.

Publication should enable comparison and learning without turning complexity into a league table. Data should be disaggregated by service type and context and accompanied by explanation of resources and population. A single ranking may encourage patient selection or under-reporting; presenting multiple dimensions supports improvement without creating an incentive to hide.

Every report should include commitments for the next year and follow-up on previous commitments. The public then sees not only what happened but what was done in response. The relevant Knesset committee should hold a public hearing, and implementing bodies should answer for gaps that remain open. Repeated reporting creates institutional memory and makes it harder to substitute a new slogan for correction.

Implementation Map for the First Five Years

Stage	**Required Output**	**Responsible Owner**	**Transition Condition**
Baseline	Uniform indicators and major disparities	Ministry of Health and participating organizations	Sufficient data quality
Pilot	Implementation in several diverse settings	Site managers and the national lead body	Improvement without material harm
Evaluation	Independent report and institutional responses	Independent evaluation body	Detailed corrective plan
Scale-up	Permanent budget, training, and information system	Government, health funds, and hospitals	Sustainable financing and operational capacity
Reassessment	Decision on continuation, modification, or termination	Legislature, regulator, and public	Publication of reasons and results

A new compact will succeed only if it replaces invisible work with visible accountability: who explains, who coordinates, who protects, who responds, and who learns. Legislation, budgets, and professional culture must move together. A program that does not define risk, cost, and stopping conditions may create one more institution; a program that is tested over time can turn rights and safety into routine practice.

Appendix A: Proposed Charter of Rights and Responsibilities for the Israeli Healthcare System

Patient Rights

1. To receive appropriate, professional, and respectful medical care without discrimination and under conditions that protect privacy as far as reasonably possible.

2. To receive clear information, adapted to language and level of understanding, about the medical condition, alternatives, risks, and likelihood of benefit.

3. To participate in decisions, consent, refuse, or request a second opinion, subject to law and emergency circumstances.

4. To review medical information, know who has accessed it, and receive an explanation of material uses of information and automated systems.

5. To submit a complaint or appeal without fear of harm to care and receive a reasoned response within a reasonable time.

Staff Rights

1. To work in a safe environment, receive protection from violence, harassment, and threats, and receive institutional backing after an incident.

2. To receive reasonable staffing, equipment, training, and time that enable safe care and proper communication.

3. To raise professional concerns and report an error or risk without retaliation, within a just culture of learning and accountability.

4. To set professional boundaries and decline an action that is not medically justified, while providing an explanation and a route for appeal.

5. To receive a fair process when a complaint is filed and to have dignity and privacy protected.

Responsibilities of Patients and the Public

1. To provide relevant information as far as possible, ask when something is not understood, and inform the team of a change in a decision.

2. To respect staff, other patients, their privacy, and reasonable safety rules.

3. To use complaint and appeal pathways and refrain from threats, violence, or attempts to obtain priority by force.

4. To notify the service of appointment cancellation when possible and use public resources responsibly, without this reducing the right to necessary care.

5. To recognize that the right to information and choice is not a right to compel treatment without a medical indication or to harm another person's rights.

Responsibilities of the State and Institutions

1. To ensure funding, planning, and staffing standards that enable realization rather than mere declaration of rights.

2. To publish waiting times, disparities, quality data, and violence data and act to correct inequality.

3. To provide interpretation, accessibility accommodations, non-digital alternatives, and a simple independent complaint mechanism.

4. To protect privacy in information systems and oversee the use of artificial intelligence and secondary-use data.

5. To involve patients and workers in planning, publish lessons from incidents, and review implementation of the charter every two years.

This charter does not derogate from the Patients' Rights Law, the National Health Insurance Law, or any other law. Its purpose is to translate their principles into a public language of compact, responsibility, and safety.

Appendix B: Framework for Assessing the Realization of Rights in a Healthcare Institution

Instructions for Using the Framework

The table is intended as a working tool rather than a one-time ranking. Each domain should be scored from 0 to 3: 0 indicates that no procedure or information exists; 1 indicates that a procedure exists but implementation is partial and unmeasured; 2 indicates regular implementation with data, but remaining gaps or variation among units; and 3 indicates consistent implementation, outcome review, and a documented corrective process. Every score should be supported by evidence rather than by a manager's general impression.

Measurement should take place at least quarterly in rapidly changing domains and at least annually in more stable domains. Before setting a target, a baseline, population, and measurement period should be documented, and at least two sources should be combined - for example, a patient survey and record review. Departments should be compared only when service type and complexity are similar, and results should always be disaggregated by language, region, and social characteristics so that an institutional average does not conceal a group left behind.

Each indicator should have a responsible owner, target, review date, and agreed response to deviation. Data should not end in a report: when a gap is found, the team should formulate a limited action, test it during a trial period, and decide whether to expand, modify, or stop it. Patient and worker representatives should be involved in selecting indicators because they may identify an outcome that looks acceptable numerically but does not reflect actual experience.

Domain	Assessment Question	Possible Indicator	Data Source
Information and consent	Did the patient understand the alternatives and material risks?	Rate of documented teach-back and an understanding measure	Patient survey and record review
Accessibility	Can the service be obtained within a reasonable time and distance?	Median waiting time and regional disparity	Scheduling systems and health-fund data
Language and culture	Was a professional interpreter offered when needed?	Use of interpretation by language	Interpretation-service log
Privacy	Did conversation and examination occur under respectful conditions?	Privacy complaints and environmental observation	Public inquiries and survey
Continuity	Did discharge include responsibility and follow-up?	Follow-up within target time and readmission	Medical record and scheduling system
Complaints	Is there a simple contact point and a timely answer?	Response time and correction rate	Inquiry system
Staff safety	Are violent incidents reported and addressed?	Reporting rate, response time, and support	Safety reports and human-resources data
Equality	Are there disparities in outcomes or access?	Gap by region, language, and social status	Disaggregated quality data
Digital information	Is use of information transparent and secure?	Access anomalies and public notifications	Access logs and privacy audit
Public participation	Did patients influence planning?	Number of processes and changes made	Protocols and management reports

How to Interpret Gaps Between Indicators

A single composite score should not be calculated if it allows a serious failure to disappear into an average. A privacy breach, lack of response to an urgent complaint, or a severe access disparity requires action even when other domains score highly. When a process indicator improves but patient experience does not - for example, more consent forms without better understanding - the institution should ask whether the indicator measures activity rather than outcome. Conversely, an increase in complaints may reflect deterioration, but it may also reflect greater trust in the complaint system; it should therefore be interpreted alongside severity, response time, and correction rate.

Once a year, a short public summary should be published: what was measured, where gaps were found, what actions were taken, and what remains incomplete. Publication should protect privacy and should not turn the framework into a marketing competition. Its purpose is to support accountability and learning over time so that the institution can demonstrate not only that it recognizes rights, but that it knows how to identify where they erode and correct the conditions that prevent their realization.

Appendix C: The Patients' Rights Law at a Glance

The table summarizes the main arrangements for orientation purposes. It does not present every provision, regulation, or judgment, does not decide an individual dispute, and does not replace legal advice. When there is medical urgency or a dispute during treatment, the treating team, institutional officer, or ethics committee should be contacted immediately as appropriate.

Topic	**Existing Law in Brief**	**Main Limit and Practical Pathway**	**Where Discussed in This Book**
Appropriate medical care	A patient is entitled to professional, quality medical care provided with proper human relations and with protection of dignity and privacy.	The meaning of 'appropriate' depends on law, professional standards, and circumstances. An immediate failure should be raised with the team and responsible officer; a recurring failure with public inquiries or the regulator.	Chapter Six; Chapter Seven
Non-discrimination	A patient may not be discriminated against in receiving medical care on prohibited grounds defined by law.	Medical distinctions based on urgency, risk, or expected benefit are not necessarily discrimination. Ask for the criterion and reasons, and document barriers of language, accessibility, or residence.	Chapter Six; Chapter Seven
Emergency care	In a medical emergency, urgent care should be provided according to capability and need without delaying life-saving treatment for administrative clarification.	After stabilization, explanation, consent, and continued-care planning should be completed. If transfer is required, the institution should support continuity and transfer necessary information.	Chapter Six
Identity of caregiver	A patient has a right	The right does not	Chapter Six; Chapter

Topic	Existing Law in Brief	Main Limit and Practical Pathway	Where Discussed in This Book
and continuity	to know who is providing care and, in appropriate circumstances, to receive continued care or referral when a caregiver or institution does not continue treatment.	guarantee a particular caregiver in every situation. It is advisable to request a name, role, contact point for continuation, and a summary document.	Seven
Second opinion	A patient may request an additional professional opinion, and the caregiver and institution are required to assist reasonably in obtaining it.	Availability, financing, and urgency may affect implementation. Request transfer of documents, clarify the medical time window, and document disagreement between opinions.	Chapter Six
Informed consent	Medical treatment requires consent based on material information concerning diagnosis, procedure, benefit, risks, alternatives, and the risk of no treatment.	A signature alone does not prove understanding. Information should be given as early as possible and in understandable language; the patient may ask questions, request time, and change a decision.	Chapters Two, Three, and Six
Treatment without consent	The law recognizes limited exceptions, including emergencies and special conditions for use of an ethics committee.	Urgency or communication difficulty should not be turned into general authorization. Capacity, accommodations, prior wishes, proportionality, and the reasons should be assessed and documented.	Chapter Six
Medical record and access	The institution must maintain a medical record, and the patient is entitled to receive medical information from it subject to statutory exceptions.	Third-party information or an exceptional risk of harm may justify a reasoned limitation. A patient may request a copy, explanation, factual correction, or addition of a position.	Chapters Three and Six

Topic	**Existing Law in Brief**	**Main Limit and Practical Pathway**	**Where Discussed in This Book**
Confidentiality and disclosure	Institutional staff must keep medical information confidential; disclosure is permitted with consent or under a legal ground.	Only information needed for the purpose should be disclosed. Authorization to a family member should be clear and revocable; an open screen or hallway conversation can also be a privacy event.	Chapters Three and Six
Ethics committee	An institutional committee is authorized to decide certain matters assigned to it by law, including exceptional situations involving treatment or disclosure of information.	The committee is not a general compensation route and does not replace a court. In an urgent dispute, review should be requested while the decision can still be changed.	Chapter Six
Complaint, review, and remedy	The response depends on the type of harm: immediate clinical resolution, public inquiries, disciplinary or regulatory review, and sometimes legal proceedings.	It is useful to define what is being requested: stopping an action, completing information, obtaining a document, apology, process correction, or compensation. Keep records and dates.	Chapters Six and Fifteen

Working rule for the reader: first determine which decision is still open, who has authority to change it, and within what timeframe. Only then choose the route of approach. This distinction prevents a long complaint from replacing an urgent solution, or a principled dispute from disappearing into a local conversation.

Appendix D: Map of Laws Related to Patients' Rights

The Patients' Rights Law is a central axis, but it does not by itself regulate every decision in the healthcare system. At times a special law adds a right, establishes a different mechanism, or permits a limited infringement of autonomy under strict conditions. The map below helps identify when the general law is not sufficient.

Related Legal Framework	**What It Regulates**	**Relationship to the Patients' Rights Law**	**Key Review Question**
National Health Insurance Law	Residency, health-fund membership, the basket of services, health-fund responsibilities, and principles of justice, equality, and mutual assistance.	The Patients' Rights Law mainly regulates the clinical encounter and process; the insurance law addresses entitlement to service and the body required to provide it.	Is the dispute about the manner of treatment, or about entitlement itself, financing, and availability?
Dying Patient Law	End-of-life decisions, the definition of a terminally ill patient, advance medical directives, and power of attorney.	This is a special framework that balances the patient's wishes, the sanctity of life, and prevention of suffering. General consent rules do not exhaust the situation.	Is the statutory definition met, and are valid directives or a registered proxy in place?
Treatment of Mentally Ill Persons Law	Psychiatric examination, hospitalization, and treatment, including coercion, psychiatric committees, and appeals.	The law permits restrictions on liberty and autonomy only under the conditions and procedures it establishes; other rights to dignity, information, and representation remain central.	Who issued the order, what is its validity, and what are the representation and appeal routes?
Legal Capacity and Guardianship Law	Legal capacity, guardianship, enduring power of attorney, and supported decision-making.	This law helps determine who makes decisions and how a person is supported, but it does not release the team from speaking with the patient and assessing capacity in	Can the person be enabled to decide through accommodation or support before moving to substituted decision-making?

Related Legal Framework	What It Regulates	Relationship to the Patients' Rights Law	Key Review Question
		relation to the specific decision.	
Protection of Privacy Law, including Amendment 13	Collection, retention, use, security, and enforcement concerning personal information and databases. Amendment 13 entered into force on 14 August 2025.	Medical confidentiality concerns disclosure within care; privacy law broadens the perspective to the data life cycle and organizational duties.	What is the purpose of the use, what is the legal basis, who may access the information, and how is data security protected?
Genetic Information Law	Genetic testing and counseling, retention of information, permitted uses, and protection against specified uses.	Genetic information may also concern relatives and therefore requires special arrangements beyond ordinary confidentiality rules.	Were appropriate explanations and counseling provided, and what will happen to the sample and information in the future?
Equal Rights for Persons with Disabilities Law and Accessibility Regulations	Physical, service, and information accessibility and equal participation of persons with disabilities.	This framework gives practical content to non-discrimination and understanding: accommodation is not a favor but a condition for realizing the right.	What accommodation is required so that the person can reach, understand, communicate, and use the service?
Anatomy and Pathology Law and Organ Transplant Law	Autopsy, use of the body after death, organ removal, allocation, and transplant controls.	These laws regulate decisions in which the patient may not be able to express a wish in real time, so consent, prior wishes, and institutional procedure take a special form.	What were the person's wishes, who is authorized to decide, and what is the precise purpose of using the body or organ?

Working Order When Laws Intersect

1. Identify the concrete decision: treatment, financing, information, coercion, representation, accessibility, or end of life.

2. Check whether a special law applies. When a special framework exists, it is read alongside the Patients' Rights Law rather than automatically replacing it.

3. Separate the existence of authority from the manner in which it is exercised. Even lawful authority requires proportionality, explanation, documentation, and review.

4. Identify the proper contact point and timeframe: treating team, institutional committee, health fund, regulator, appeal committee, or court - according to the type of decision and its urgency.

Source Note and Edition Update

The bibliographic sources, foundational documents, and legal materials cited in this book reflect information available during preparation of this edition through July 2026. References in the body are intended to direct readers to principal sources without overloading the flow of reading, and the bibliography below supports further inquiry. Legislation, case law, procedures, and public policy may change after this date; the book offers historical, ethical, and comparative analysis and is not a substitute for individualized legal or clinical advice.

Chapter-by-Chapter Source Guide

This guide points to anchor sources for verification and further study. It does not replace references within the chapters or the complete bibliography.

Chapter	**Primary or Institutional Sources**	**Key Interpretive Sources**
One	Hippocratic Oath; writings of Maimonides and the medical tradition	Edelstein; Rosner; Kleinman
Two	Nuremberg Code; Declaration of Helsinki; Belmont Report	Faden & Beauchamp; Jonsen
Three	Human-rights instruments; privacy and ethics documents	Beauchamp & Childress; O'Neill; Mol; Elwyn et al.
Four	Israeli health-system documents and early legislation	Rothman; literature on institutions, professionalism, and the welfare state
Five	Basic Law: Human Dignity and Liberty; National Health Insurance Law; Patients' Rights Bill	Israeli case law and literature on the transition from professional discourse to rights discourse
Six	Patients' Rights Law; the Reibi, Vaturi, Daaka, Stendel, and Sidi	Literature on informed consent, autonomy, and shared decision-making

Chapter	**Primary or Institutional Sources**	**Key Interpretive Sources**
	judgments	
Seven	Ministry of Health and State Comptroller reports and quality and accessibility data	Institute of Medicine; WHO; Marmot
Eight	Ministry of Health circulars and research reports on violence in the healthcare system	WHO/ILO/ICN/PSI; Brookdale studies
Nine	Data on violence, complaints, burnout, and policy documents	Methodological literature on causality, organization, and trust
Ten	Constitutions of Brazil and Bolivia; PAHO documents	Literature on constitutional rights, decentralization, and intercultural health
Eleven	EMTALA; Canada Health Act; CMS guidance	Literature on insurance coverage, equality, and access
Twelve	Thai laws; WHO, NHSO, Japan, and Malaysia documents	Health-system reviews and literature on culture, end of life, and compensation
Thirteen	Nigerian laws; Constitution of South Africa; Treatment Action Campaign	Literature on progressive realization, scarcity, and distributive justice
Fourteen	NHS Constitution; German and European Observatory documents	Welfare-state reviews, self-governance, and ombudsman literature
Fifteen	Legislation and reports discussed throughout the book	Daniels; Yamin; Gostin; WHO patient-safety materials

Bibliography

Scholarly Literature

Bayer, R., & Fairchild, A. L. (2004). The genesis of public health ethics. Bioethics, 18(6), 473-492. doi: 10.1111/j.1467-8519.2004.00412.x

Beauchamp, T. L., & Childress, J. F. (2019). Principles of Biomedical Ethics (8th ed.). Oxford University Press.

Daniels, N. (2008). Just Health: Meeting Health Needs Fairly. Cambridge University Press.

Edelstein, L. (1943). The Hippocratic Oath: Text, Translation, and Interpretation. Johns Hopkins Press.

Elwyn, G., Frosch, D., Thomson, R., Joseph-Williams, N., Lloyd, A., Kinnersley, P., Cording, E., Tomson, D., Dodd, C., Rollnick, S., Edwards, A., & Barry, M. (2012). Shared decision making: A model for clinical practice. Journal of General Internal Medicine, 27(10), 1361-1367. doi: 10.1007/s11606-012-2077-6

Elwyn, G., Durand, M.-A., Song, J., Aarts, J., Barr, P. J., Berger, Z., Cochran, N., Frosch, D., Galasiński, D., Gulbrandsen, P., Han, P. K. J., Härter, M., Kinnersley, P., Lloyd, A., Mishra, M., Perestelo-Perez, L., Scholl, I., Tomori, K., Trevena, L., Witteman, H. O., & Van der Weijden, T. (2017). A three-talk model for shared decision making: Multistage consultation process. BMJ, 359, j4891. doi: 10.1136/bmj.j4891

Faden, R. R., & Beauchamp, T. L. (1986). A History and Theory of Informed Consent. Oxford University Press.

Gostin, L. O. (2014). Global Health Law. Harvard University Press.

Institute of Medicine. (2000). To Err Is Human: Building a Safer Health System. National Academies Press. doi: 10.17226/9728

Jonsen, A. R. (1998). The Birth of Bioethics. Oxford University Press.

Kleinman, A. (1988). The Illness Narratives: Suffering, Healing, and the Human Condition. Basic Books.

Marmot, M. (2015). The Health Gap: The Challenge of an Unequal World. Bloomsbury.

Mol, A. (2008). The Logic of Care: Health and the Problem of Patient Choice. Routledge. doi: 10.4324/9780203927076

O'Neill, O. (2002). Autonomy and Trust in Bioethics. Cambridge University Press.

Rosner, F. (1998). The Medical Legacy of Moses Maimonides. KTAV Publishing House.

Rothman, D. J. (2003). Strangers at the Bedside: A History of How Law and Bioethics Transformed Medical Decision Making (2nd pbk. ed.). Aldine de Gruyter.

Sen, A. (1999). Development as Freedom. Alfred A. Knopf.

Yamin, A. E. (2023). When Misfortune Becomes Injustice: Evolving Human Rights Struggles for Health and Social Equality (2nd ed.). Stanford University Press.

Foundational Documents, Ethics, and Medical Research

National Commission for the Protection of Human Subjects of Biomedical and Behavioral Research. (1979). The Belmont Report. U.S. Department of Health and Human Services.

United Nations Committee on Economic, Social and Cultural Rights. (2000). General Comment No. 14: The Right to the Highest Attainable Standard of Health (E/C.12/2000/4).

United Nations. (1966). International Covenant on Economic, Social and Cultural Rights, Article 12.

UNESCO. (2005). Universal Declaration on Bioethics and Human Rights.

United States v. Brandt et al. (1947). Nuremberg Code: Directives for Human Experimentation.

World Medical Association. (2024). Declaration of Helsinki: Ethical Principles for Medical Research Involving Human Participants.

World Health Organization. (1946). Constitution of the World Health Organization.

World Health Organization. (2017). Advancing the Right to Health: The Vital Role of Law.

World Health Organization. (2021). Global Patient Safety Action Plan 2021-2030: Towards Eliminating Avoidable Harm in Health Care.

World Health Organization, International Labour Organization, International Council of Nurses, & Public Services International. (2002). Framework Guidelines for Addressing Workplace Violence in the Health Sector.

Israeli Legislation, Case Law, and Reports

Basic Law: Human Dignity and Liberty, 5752-1992.

National Health Insurance Law, 5754-1994, Sefer HaHukkim 1469, p. 156.

Patients' Rights Law, 5756-1996, Sefer HaHukkim 1591, p. 327.

Knesset. (1992). Patients' Rights Bill, 5752-1992, H.H. 2132.

Office of the State Comptroller. (2015). Protecting the Rights and Dignity of Hospitalized Patients. Annual Report 65C.

Ministry of Health. (2006). The Patient Rights Charter: A Decade after the Patients' Rights Law. Director-General Circular 9/06.

Ministry of Health. (2020). Preparedness for the Prevention and Management of Violence in the Healthcare System. Director-General Circular 6/2020.

Blumenthal, A., Senior, A., Elizra, R., et al. (2021). Violence Toward Staff in Community Clinics: Research Report. Myers-JDC-Brookdale Institute and Ministry of Health.

Myers-JDC-Brookdale Institute & Ministry of Health. (2023). The National Program to Reduce Violence Against Medical Staff in Hospitals: Evaluation Study.

CA 3108/91 Reibi v. Veigel, PD 47(2) 497 (1993).

CA 4384/90 Vaturi v. Laniado Hospital, PD 51(2) 171 (1997).

CA 2781/93 Daaka v. Carmel Hospital, PD 53(4) 526 (1999).

CA 6153/97 Stendel v. Prof. Sadeh, PD 56(4) 746 (2002).

CA 4960/04 Sidi v. General Federation Health Fund, PD 60(3) 590 (2005).

Ministry of Health. (2024). Protecting Patient Privacy in the Digital Transmission of Medical Information.

Privacy Protection Authority & Ministry of Health. (2026). Professional Guide to Anonymization of Medical Information.

Anatomy and Pathology Law, 5713-1953; Organ Transplant Law, 5768-2008.

Equal Rights for Persons with Disabilities Law, 5758-1998; Equal Rights for Persons with Disabilities (Accessibility Adjustments to Health Services and Places Where They Are Provided) Regulations, 5776-2016.

Genetic Information Law, 5761-2000.

Protection of Privacy Law, 5741-1981, including Amendment No. 13, 5784-2024, effective 14 August 2025.

Legal Capacity and Guardianship Law, 5722-1962, including Amendment No. 18, 5776-2016.

Treatment of Mentally Ill Persons Law, 5751-1991.

Dying Patient Law, 5766-2005, Sefer HaHukkim 2039, p. 58.

Comparative Sources: The Americas, Asia, Africa, and Europe

Brazil. (1988). Constitution of the Federative Republic of Brazil, arts. 196-200.

Bolivia. (2009). Political Constitution of the Plurinational State of Bolivia.

Canada. (1985). Canada Health Act, R.S.C. 1985, c. C-6.

Centers for Medicare & Medicaid Services. (2026). Emergency Medical Treatment & Labor Act (EMTALA): Statute and Interpretive Guidance.

United States. Emergency Medical Treatment and Labor Act, 42 U.S.C. § 1395dd.

Pan American Health Organization. (2022). Health in the Americas: Bolivia Country Profile.

Pan American Health Organization. (2022). Health in the Americas: Brazil Country Profile and materials on the Sistema Único de Saúde.

Thailand. (2002). National Health Security Act, B.E. 2545, section 41.

Thailand. (2007). National Health Act, B.E. 2550, section 12.

National Health Security Office of Thailand. (2022). Health System Responsiveness and Rights Protection under the Universal Coverage Scheme.

World Health Organization. (2019). UHC Law in Practice: Legal Access Rights to Health Care-Country Profiles: Germany, Japan, Kenya and Thailand.

Malaysian Medical Council. (2019). Code of Professional Conduct.

Malaysian Medical Council. (2025). Consent for Treatment of Patients by Registered Medical Practitioners.

Ministry of Health Malaysia. (2023). Health White Paper for Malaysia.

Ministry of Health Malaysia. (2024). Advance Care Planning: A Guide for Healthcare Practitioners in Malaysia.

Malaysia. (1998). Private Healthcare Facilities and Services Act 1998, with Regulations 2006.

Nigeria. (2014). National Health Act 2014.

Nigeria. (2022). National Health Insurance Authority Act 2022.

South Africa. (1996). Constitution of the Republic of South Africa, section 27.

South Africa. (2003). National Health Act 61 of 2003.

Minister of Health v. Treatment Action Campaign (No. 2) 2002 (5) SA 721 (CC).

Department of Health and Social Care. (2023). The NHS Constitution for England.

Department of Health and Social Care. (2023). Handbook to the NHS Constitution for England.

European Observatory on Health Systems and Policies. (2020). Germany: Health System Review. Health Systems in Transition.

World Health Organization. (2018). Japan Health System Review. Health Systems in Transition.

Subject Index

The index points to pages where the concept is discussed substantively, rather than to every incidental occurrence.

Index of Legislation, Case Law, and Foundational Documents

Alongside Israeli legislation, this index includes international instruments and major judgments discussed in the book.

www.ingramcontent.com/pod-product-compliance
Lightning Source LLC
LaVergne TN
LVHW010714061126
851857LV00014B/1174

* 9 7 8 9 6 5 9 3 3 9 7 0 9 *